HUMAN BRAINWAVES

This book is dedicated to the memory of my father, the poet
William Empson.

HUMAN BRAINWAVES
The Psychological Significance of the Electroencephalogram

Jacob Empson

Department of Psychology
The University, Hull HU6 7RX, UK

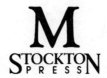

First published 1986

Published in the United Kingdom by
THE MACMILLAN PRESS LTD
Houndmills, Basingstoke, Hampshire RG21 2XS
and London
Companies and representatives
throughout the world

Printed in Great Britain by
The Camelot Press Ltd,
Southampton

British Library Cataloguing in Publication Data
Empson, Jacob A. C.
Human brainwaves : the psychological significance
of the electroencephalogram.
1. Electroencephalography
I. Title
616.8'047547   RC386.6.E43
ISBN 0–333–41354–7
ISBN 0–333–41355–5 Pbk

Published in the United States and Canada, 1986, by
Stockton Press
15 East 26th Street, New York, NY 10010

Library of Congress Cataloging-in-Publication Data
Empson, Jacob, 1944–
Human brainwaves
1. Electroencephalography. 2. Neuropsychology –
Technique. 3. Sleep – Physiological aspects I. Title
QP 360.E47 1986   612'.82   86–5987
ISBN 0–947818–92–3

Contents

Preface

This book is addressed to students of psychology and others interested in the latest advances in the cognitive neurosciences. It deals with contemporary attempts by encephalographers to resolve problems in cognitive psychology, outlining the contributions that the EEG has made in topics such as sleep and dreaming, meditation, biofeedback, attentional processes and hemispheric lateralisation.

Much of what we know about brainwaves was established in the 1930s, and the story of psychological research in subsequent years was largely one of disappointment in this promising new technique, although it found a role as a useful clinical instrument for neurologists. A notable exception, and perhaps still the greatest achievement of electrophysiology for psychology, was the identification of the mechanisms subserving the control of activation in the brain, and the use of EEG in assessing level of arousal.

In the more recent past, however, the advent of new methods of data processing with computers has revolutionised our old EEG machines. Frequency analysis and the averaging of event-related potentials have provided powerful tools in the analysis of cognitive processes. In addition, the combination of EEG with other psychophysiological measures — eye movements (EOG) and muscle activity (EMG) — has given us entirely novel methods for scoring sleep stages in human subjects. Sleep stage analysis has become crucial to our understanding of the rhythms of sleep and of its functions.

EEG techniques involve some formidable-looking equipment, and the addition of computers to the EEG laboratory has only increased its 'high-tech', incomprehensible and highly impressive appearance to the outsider. Some areas of research — such as the analysis of cognitive processes using event-related potentials — have actually become so impenetrable that only a small band of people seem to understand them. This book attempts to make this arcane world accessible. The historical account of the development of electrophysiological techniques is intrinsically fascinating and also provides a relatively non-technical introduction to the EEG. The practical guide to recording procedures should also help demystify the subject.

I was helped and encouraged by many people in the writing of this book; and I would particularly like to thank my friend Ray Meddis for his supportive criticisms of some early drafts and his advice on the sleep chapters, Tony Gaillard for generously putting me on the right lines on event-related potentials, and Sam Connally for his comments on meditation and biofeedback. Invaluable practical help from my students John McKeown and Jorge Da Silva is also gratefully acknowledged. The book was entirely written on a Sinclair QL microcomputer, whose reputation for the calamitous discombobulation of data files provided a continual *frisson* of danger.

Hull, 1985 J.A.C.E.

1

The History and Origin of the EEG

HISTORY OF THE EEG

The development of encephalography, like that of all other electrophysiological techniques, was dependent on advances in the science of electromagnetism finding appropriate applications in the mid- to late nineteenth century. However, there were one or two early attempts to investigate the relationship between electricity and living organisms during the eighteenth century, long before the technology existed to do so properly. According to Grey Walter in his book *The Living Brain* (Walter, 1953), informal experiments on executed criminals showed that electric shocks caused muscles to contract and twitch, and Louis XV 'caused an electric shock from a battery of Leyden jars to be administered to 700 Carthusian monks joined hand to hand, with prodigious effect'. The Leyden jar was simply a primitive condenser, capable of storing static electricity for short periods of time, and more refined experiments had to await the invention of reliable sources of electric current.

In fact, it is said that the claims about the electrical nature of living processes made by the Galvanis in 1791 stimulated Volta into inventing the first battery cell. This consisted of silver or copper alternating with zinc plates, separated by flannel soaked in brine, and it became known as the Voltaic pile. Luigi and Lucia Galvani had begun their work from observations of the convulsive movements of a dead frog, hung from an iron balustrade by a copper wire during a thunderstorm. They became convinced that they had proved that nerves contained an intrinsic form of electricity. Volta repeated their experiments, but showed that electricity could be generated without the frog, or a storm, merely by the presence of two metals and a conducting solution, forming a simple electrical cell. The movements of the Galvanis' frog had presumably been caused by the resultant electrical stimulation.

Electrical stimulation could produce dramatic effects, but the proper study of electrophysiology had to wait for some time until it was possible to record small electrical potentials. The gold leaf electroscope, available early in the nineteenth century, was too insensitive to register the tiny changes in potential differences associated with nervous and muscular activity.

However, Volta's invention provided a reliable source of steady current, which allowed of the development and elaboration of electromagnetic principles. By 1820 H.C. Oersted and A.M. Ampère had described the magnetic field that surrounds a conductor carrying an electric current, and quantified the relationship between the strength of the field and that of the current producing it. It was not until 1831 that this knowledge was applied, by Faraday. He showed that a simple application of this principle allowed of the conversion of mechanical into electrical power, and the reverse. This insight into the possibilities offered by a known scientific principle was the cornerstone of the new science of electro-magnetism. It allowed of the immediate development of sensitive electrical instruments, such as the string galvanometer, which was standard equipment for the early electroencephalographers.

Essentially, the string galvanometer consisted of a coil of copper wire, connected at either end to two electrodes, and string hanging down within the coil to which was attached a small magnetised mirror. A difference in electrical potential between the two electrodes would cause a current flow through the coil, creating a magnetic field within. The mirror would then rotate in proportion to the strength of the current. A light, shone onto the mirror and reflected onto a fairly distant surface, would provide an initial doubling in amplification of the movement of the mirror, and the further the light was projected the greater the subsequent amplification. One way of obtaining a permanent record, in the nineteenth century, was for one observer to watch the galvanometer mirror through a telescope and work a key with his finger which operated a signal pen on a smoked drum kymograph. The magnitude of excursion of the mirror was read aloud by a second observer (watching the projected light) to an assistant who wrote on the drum next to the appropriate signal.

Despite these enormous difficulties in recording electrical changes in living tissue, Du Bois-Reymond, working in Berlin in 1848, had discovered the standing potential between the surface and the cut end of a nerve, and also the sudden negative variation in response to a stimulus, now known as the 'action potential'. He must be regarded as the founding father of electrophysiology: apart from being a very important innovator, he was also a long-lived teacher, with many distinguished pupils, such as Sechenov, the great Russian physiologist. To quote Du Bois-Reymond in 1848: 'If I do not greatly deceive myself, I have succeeded in realising (albeit under a slightly different aspect) the hundred years' dream of physicists and physiologists, to wit, the identification of the nervous principle with electricity.'

The apparatus and techniques now existed to record from animals' brains, and also to stimulate living preparations. An apparently apocryphal account is of two Prussian medical officers, Fritsch and Hitzig, who in 1870 took advantage of the opportunity offered by the Franco–Prussian War to study the exposed brains of soldiers struck down on the battlefield. What is certain is that they discovered that Galvanic stimulation of some parts of the cortex caused movements in the contralateral limbs, and that these movements could be reliably elicited by stimulation at the same place. Whether it was a dog acting as the subject for this experiment on the kitchen table (according to Brazier, 1961) or a dog in Hitzig's wife's bedroom, lightly anaesthetised (according to Nathan, 1969), is unimportant. It was now possible to map what we now know as the motor cortex in terms of the musculature it controlled, and this Fritsch and Hitzig did in the dog and in the monkey. The procedure, incidentally, was not as cruel as it may sound, as the surface of the brain is totally insensitive: operations on the brain in humans commonly involve only a local anaesthetic, with the patient conscious and reporting to the surgeon on any experiences he or she may be having as the operation progresses.

It was now obvious that with sufficiently sensitive recording techniques it should be possible to map the sensory cortex in a similar way. This was the task that Richard Caton, working in Liverpool, set himself, using a Thomson reflecting galvanometer and Du Bois-Reymond's coated, non-polarisable electrodes. Caton repeated some of Du Bois-Reymond's early experiments on the electrophysiology of nerve and muscle preparations, and then set about recording from the exposed surface of the brains of living rabbits and monkeys. He demonstrated his findings at a meeting of the British Medical Association on 24 August 1875 in Edinburgh, and a report of the demonstration was published in the *British Medical Journal* (Caton, 1875): 'In every brain hitherto examined, the galvanometer has indicated the existence of electric currents. The external surface of the grey matter is usually positive in relation to the surface of a section through it. Feeble currents of varying direction pass through the multiplier when the electrodes are on two points of the external surface. . .' He had thus discovered spontaneous EEG in animals, and also showed that it was indeed possible to detect electrical brain responses to stimuli and located the visual cortex in the occiput, or rear of the head. He was unable to find any location specifically responsive to sound stimulation. The observation that there was spontaneous electrical activity at the surface of the cortex seemed relatively insignificant at the time, but it was the discovery of the electroencephalogram.

At that time there was no British journal of physiology, so all Caton's work was published in medical journals. It may be for this reason that his papers were not widely read, and were unknown to Continental physiologists. Adolf Beck, a Polish scientist, presented his doctoral thesis on the electrical activity of the brain in 1890, completely unaware of Caton's work (Beck, 1890). He had unknowingly repeated many of Caton's experiments, as well as recording spontaneous oscillations in potential from the occipital cortex. He also found that this occipital oscillation disappeared with light stimulation (using a magnesium flare) but not with noise. (This seems analogous with the phenomenon of alpha blocking found in humans 40 years later.)

Beck was doubly anticipated, since, once he had published his findings, a German, Fleischl von Marxow (1890), revealed that he, too, had made similar observations and had deposited a sealed letter 7 years before with the Imperial Academy of Sciences in Vienna! Presumably, the lack of any method of producing a permanent record of the potentials might have exposed any scientist making these sorts of claims to ridicule and derision, and von Marxow was too sensitive to brave this possibility. Yet another Continental, Vasili Danilevsky, had been working on brain potentials prior to this (in 1876) and had also noticed the spontaneous activity produced by the resting cortex, but he had not published his work, which was deposited as a thesis of the University of Kharkov in 1877.

Many of the techniques and practices were crude in the extreme, and it is not surprising that scientists had some reservations about the significance of the spontaneous oscillations in the minute currents that were being recorded, even to the extent of showing some reluctance to publish. The spontaneous electrical activity shown by the cortex could only be regarded as a curiosity while there was no way of making a permanent record of any sort. It was technically feasible to make a photographic record, but few laboratories could afford the specialised cameras. Beck, for instance, wrote: 'All these changes could be easily and nicely presented in a graphical form with the help of a galvanometer with a photographic attachment; unfortunately our Institute does not have one, and there is no hope that it will have one in the near future.' The first photographically recorded brainwaves (of a dog) were published in 1913 by a Russian called Vladimir Vladimirovich Pravdich-Neminsky.

In her definitive monograph on the history of electroencephalography, to which this short account owes a great deal, Mary A.B. Brazier describes the work of Hans Berger as the triumph of a man working with equipment inadequate even by the standards of his day. Like Caton, Berger attempted to record electrical responses to sensory stimuli in animals, although it seems that the work he did between 1902 and 1910 was, in general, unsuccessful. It was not until 1924 that he turned to the measurement of human electrical potentials, and he delayed publication until 1929, when the first recorded electroencephalogram (of his young son) appeared in *Archiv für Psychiatrie* and Nervenkrankheiten (see Figure 1.1).

Berger discovered the alpha rhythm, running at 10 cycles per second (Hz), and also discovered that it disappeared if the eyes were opened, with mental effort (such as doing mental arithmetic with eyes closed) and with loud noises or painful stimuli.

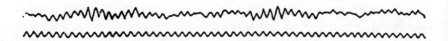

Figure 1.1 The first recorded electroencephalogram of man. The lower line is a 10 cycles per second sine wave for use as a time marker; the upper line is the recording from Berger's young son made in 1925. From Brazier (1961)

Berger's work was disregarded by physiologists, partly because it was published in psychiatric journals, and also perhaps because of his reputation for eccentricity, seclusiveness and his outstanding belief in psychic phenomena such as telepathy. Only after his work was replicated by Adrian and Matthews (1934) in Cambridge did he get the credit he deserved, for having laid the foundations of human electroencephalography.

MODERN ENCEPHALOGRAPHIC TECHNIQUES – A PRACTICAL GUIDE

The modern clinical EEG machine is a far cry from the string galvanometer devices used by Berger and the other pioneers. Entirely electronic amplifiers are arranged in banks, so that between 8 and 16 channels of EEG are transmitted to a bank of galvanometers. The use of multiple recordings has allowed of the development of a series of techniques for localising sources of electrical activity within the cranium.

Any serious application of the EEG requires a rigorous mapping of the scalp, so that the subsequent recordings of *montages* of derivations can be related to locations within the head. The standard method for electrode localisation is the so-called 10–20 electrode system, devised by H. H. Jasper in 1952 (Jasper, 1958). This system identifies 19 locations on the scalp, which relate in a proportional way to 4 reference points – the bridge of the nose (the nasion), the bump at the back of the head immediately above the neck (the inion), and the left and right preauricular points (depressions above the angle of the cheekbone just in front of the ear). The locations are labelled with letters of the alphabet (C for central, F for frontal, P for parietal and T for temporal) and numbers, odd on the left and even on the right, which generally become larger as they get further from the midline. (See Figure 1.2.) Heads vary in size and proportions, and the advantage of this system is that it accommodates practically everybody. Reference should be made to Jasper's original paper for a definitive account of the system, but the following series of rules should allow of the localisation of most points.

(1) Find the vertex (Cz). This is the point half-way between nasion and inion, and half-way between the preauricular points, in the midline.

(2) The other two midline locations (Fz and Pz) are 20 per cent of the anteriorposterior distance in front of and behind the vertex.

(3) C3 and C4 are 20 per cent of the interauricular distance to the left and right of the vertex, respectively, on the interauricular line, and T3 and T4 are 40 per cent of the interauricular distance to the left and right of the vertex.

(4) F3 and F4 are 20 per cent of the interauricular distance left and right of Fz, and P3 and P4 are a similar distance left and right of Pz.

(5) The occipital placements, O1 and O2, are 10 per cent up from the inion, and the same distance left and right of the midline.

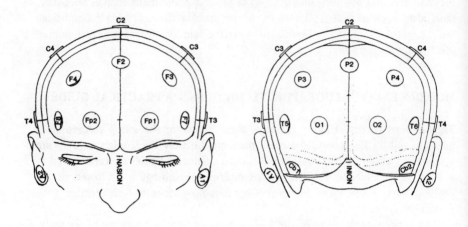

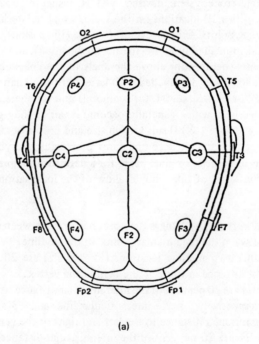

(a)

Figure 1.2 (*continued opposite*) The 10–20 system of electrode localisation. From Jasper (1958)

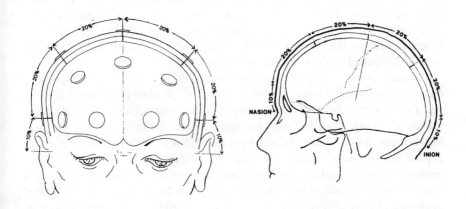

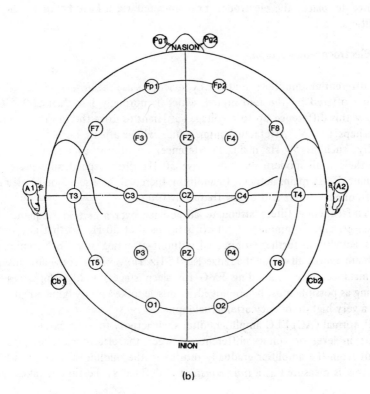

(b)

Electrodes

EEG electrodes are made of silver and coated with silver chloride. They may either be circular, dished and directly attached to a lead, or be encased in a cotton-wool wad. The former are attached to the scalp with glue (collodion); the latter are held on the scalp by a rubber-band skull-cap which does up under the chin, and attached to the wire leads with crocodile clips.

In order to ensure a good electrical connection, it is necessary to thoroughly clean the skin with a tissue soaked with alcohol or acetone. (Care should be taken not to let either of these solvents come into contact with the eyes.) When the small circular disc electrodes are used, a small quantity of electrode paste between the electrode and the skin gives a low-resistance connection, and glue is applied *above* the electrode, normally by draping some hair over it before applying the glue. Glued-on electrodes can be removed with the help of acetone, which dissolves collodion with the help of some rubbing. Again, do not allow it to come into contact with the eyes. Electrodes are attached to hairless areas with small circular double-sided sticky discs with holes in the middle, or tape, or both. Zinc oxide tape should be avoided if possible, as it leaves red weals on the skin of some subjects. Micropore surgical tape is non-allergenic and also relatively moisture-resistant.

Once in place, the electrodes are connected via a head-board to the EEG amplifiers.

The Electroencephalograph

The differential amplifiers used in EEG machines use the *difference* between the voltages offered by the two inputs, which is normally less than 200 μV, and amplify this difference up to a voltage sufficient to drive the galvanometer pens — perhaps 0-5 V. Artefactual interference which affects both the electrodes equally, such as 50 Hz mains interference, ought not to affect the output. Nevertheless, all modern machines have 50 Hz filters, specifically designed to eliminate 50 Hz mains activity. In addition, there will be a selection of electronic high-frequency filters and of low-frequency filters.

High-frequency filters attenuate all activity over a certain frequency band non-selectively. Commonly, a cut-off is imposed at 30 Hz, so that any residual mains activity is further attenuated without affecting any EEG components, which are almost all within the range 1.5-15 Hz. However, in some circumstances (for instance, when recording EMG for sleep stages) as little high-frequency filtering as possible must be employed, as muscle spike activity is indistinguishable from a very-high-frequency artefactual input.

All normal (AC) EEG amplifiers filter slow activity to some extent. That is, if a shift in level of voltage difference between the electrodes takes place, the output from the amplifier gradually returns to the midline. The rate at which it does this is measured as a *time constant* — defined as the time it takes for the output to return 63 per cent of the way to baseline, after a shift in input voltage level. The shorter the time constant the more attenuated slow activity will be. For EEG work, it is normal to use time constants of 0.3 or 0.6 s. The EEG is thus not a reflection of the potential difference between two electrode placements, but of the *changes* in voltage taking place between them. If slow event-related potentials are being recorded, it is obviously important to use as long a time constant as possible — 1.2 s or longer. Direct-coupled (DC) recordings (where the output always refers directly to the input voltage difference, with no filtering) is rarely attempted, and is fraught with problems of voltage drift and consequent limiting at either the top or the bottom of the range of voltage output possible from a particular device.

Outputs from the banks of amplifiers drive the galvanometers which work the pens up and down. It is also increasingly usual to be able to take outputs from the final amplifiers from a series of sockets for storage on FM tape recorders, or for immediate, on-line analysis by computer. This facility is essential for most experimental work, including frequency analysis and event-related potential measurement. Figure 1.3 shows a standard eight-channel clinical EEG machine, with traces from four channels being drawn from four amplifiers whose outputs are also available through jackplug sockets (shown leading into sockets on the wall behind) for storage on magnetic tape or for immediate, 'on-line' analysis by computer.

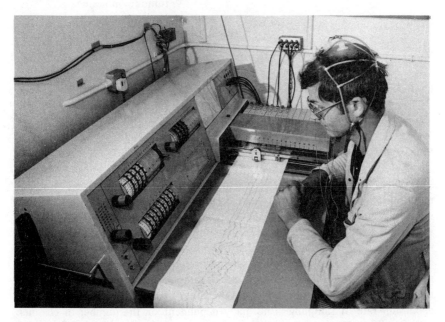

Figure 1.3 Photograph of an Elema-Schonander clinical electroencephalograph, adapted to provide outputs from four of its eight amplifiers. The elastic cap worn by the author, seated in front of the machine, is used to hold electrodes on the scalp

The Electroencephalogram

The electroencephalogram (EEG) is a mixed-frequency signal recorded from the scalp. The nomenclature in Table 1.1 is entirely descriptive, and follows a convention which is rather the result of the historical order in which the rhythms were noticed than of any more rational ordering. Rhythmic activity is defined in terms of its frequency in cycles per second, or as it is conventionally expressed, Hz.

Table 1.1

Name	Defining frequencies	Principal characteristics
Alpha	8–12 Hz	Dominates occipital scalp when eyes closed, relaxed
Beta	13<Hz	Precentral, frontal, rare except during sleep (13–15 Hz spindles) or with barbiturates
Theta	4–7 Hz	Young children, and normal adults during light sleep. Clinically, typical of space-occupying foreign bodies or tumours in brain
Delta	0.5–3.5 Hz	Ubiquitous on scalp during deep (stage 4) sleep
Mu	7–11 Hz	Central, left and right, blocked by contralateral movement
Lambda	Sharp waves	Low-amplitude single spikey waves, sometimes in association with visual stimulation

Computer Hardware

Almost all of the experiments described in this book involve the use of a computer in one form or another. An essential input device for the analysis of electrophysiological signals is the analogue–digital converter (ADC), which samples the voltage input offered by the amplifier, ascribing numbers to the values obtained. Once it has been digitised, the EEG signal can be treated by the computer as a series of numbers, and subsequent analyses are entirely on a numerical basis. Factors limiting the rate of sampling and the level of discrimination achieved can be intrinsic to the ADC rather than the central processor. The maximum rate of sampling is normally dependent on the number of channels being simultaneously dealt with. When digitised, the voltage is defined as either an 8-, 12- or 16-bit number, depending on the capacity of the ADC. The greater the number of bits used the greater the degree of discrimination it is possible to achieve. For instance, if the input voltage varies between plus and minus 2.5 V, the theoretical limit (with perfect matching of input devices) for an 8-bit ADC is to express the voltage in 5/256, or 20 mV, steps, while a 12-bit device will have a limit of discriminability of 5/4096, or 1.25 mV, steps. Highly popular machines in this connection have been the Digital Equipment Corporation's range of PDP computers, which were specifically designed in the 1960s and 1970s with the requirements of the electrophysiological laboratory in mind. The PDP LAB8e computer, for instance, which is still in use in Hull University's Psychology Department, is equipped as standard to deal with four 12-bit ADC input channels.

Frequency Analysis

The traditional method for EEG analysis has been careful visual inspection. The EEG correlates of sleep, coma or anaesthesia, for instance, are easily recognised, and there are well-recognised procedures for visual analysis of sleep records which cannot easily be duplicated by computers. Similarly, the clinician's trained eye is adept at identifying signs and patterns such as 4 Hz theta or spike and wave activity. Human perceptual abilities allow us to detect gross changes in frequency, and particular patterns, such as the K complexes of sleep, 'saw-toothed' waves or the spikes typical of epilepsy. They do not allow of accurate quantitative assessments of frequencies, especially when frequencies are mixed, as is usually the case in EEG.

Mathematicians tell us that any number series representing a waveform can be defined in terms of a number of sine wave components, which, if added together, would give the original pattern. The formal description of a waveform in these terms, Fourier analysis, is the basis of most computer-based EEG frequency analysis techniques. An alternative method is to pass the EEG signal to a series of electronic filters set at particular bands, which will indicate how much of the waveform is attributable to activity within their waveband.

Figure 1.4 shows a sample of EEG, and the outcome of analysis by a spectral analysis program. The amount of activity at every frequency between 1 and 32 Hz is represented in terms of its 'power' — an interval scale expressed in arbitrary units. The graph as a whole is therefore called a power spectrum. This particular program, one of Digital Equipment's range supplied with their PDP LAB8e, used the fast Fourier transform (FFT), an algorithmic procedure which gives an approximation of Fourier analysis. (Full Fourier analysis is very laborious computationally, and is not normally feasible as an on-line technique, even using fast modern computers.) The sampling rate was 64 Hz.

This sort of analysis allows of the objective quantification of the EEG within particular frequency bands (for instance, the alpha band, between 8 and 11 Hz) and therefore the comparison of activity between different scalp locations or between different experimental conditions. It has also been used in the objective scoring of sleep records, although not entirely successfully, as EEG is not the only measure normally used in the definition of sleep stages — electromyography

(EMG) and electro-oculography (EOG), measuring muscle activity and eye movement, are also used. (See Chapter 5 for a description of sleep-stage scoring techniques.)

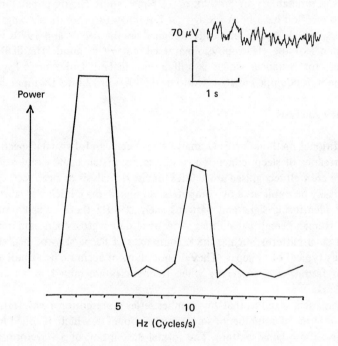

Figure 1.4 Spectral analysis of a sample of EEG, using a fast Fourier transform (FFT) procedure. This power spectrum illustrates the potential of the technique for quantifying the contribution of sine waves of different frequency to a complex waveform

Event-related Averaging

At its simplest, event-related averaging achieves no more than what Caton attempted in 1875 — to record the EEG response of the brain to a stimulus. The difficulty inherent in doing this is that much of the electrical activity recordable from the scalp will be irrelevant to the stimulus, and the EEG response to the stimulus will be buried within this noise. In order to extract the EEG activity relevant to the stimulus, repeated presentations are made and the EEG activity to all of them is digitised and summed. The resultant averaged evoked potential is then treated as the average of the components of the EEG relevant to the stimulus.

Event-related averaging techniques have been highly successful in identifying EEG components with psychological phenomena. Chapter 3 is an extended account of much of this research: to anticipate the explanations given there, Figure 1.5 shows an event-related potential to an auditory stimulus. Specialised equipment is, of course, ideal for this sort of work, but quite adequate event-related potentials can be recorded simply with a cheap microcomputer. In order to demonstrate this, the example given in Figure 1.5 was averaged on a BBC model B machine, which presented the stimuli and recorded the EEG potentials through its own ADC — normally used for operating games paddles and joysticks. The program employed, written entirely in BASIC, is given in the Appendix. While relatively inexpensive peripherals can allow of fast sampling, this machine's limitations, as it stands, for this application are that its sampling rate is relatively slow (with a maximum rate of about 120 Hz) and that the ADC itself, although nominally 12-bit, is by the manufacturers' own account best regarded as a 10-bit device. In addition, the output from the EEG amplifier (typically varying between −2.5 and +2.5 V) must be attenuated and shifted so that it varies between 0 and +1.8 V. A final word of caution: if any reader attempts to use a BBC for averaging EEG signals, it is wise to install a voltage limiter such as a Zener protector at the input side, since, unlike in many electronic devices, the voltage limiter is not already there to protect the circuitry. Inadvertently pre-senting this machine with more than about 2.5 V burns out the ADC chip!

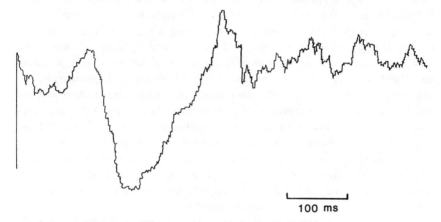

100 ms

Figure 1.5 An auditory evoked potential (40 sweeps). Recorded from Cz (the vertex) with reference to linked electrodes on the left and right mastoids, the deflection from top to bottom is of the order of 5 µV, with negative up, positive down

ORIGIN OF THE EEG

There have always been some doubts about whether the EEG actually originated in the cortex. Berger himself shared this scepticism. Recording from the scalps of patients with trephined holes in the skull, he found that the alpha rhythm was always greater when one of the electrodes was placed over the hole, and greatest when a needle electrode pierced the scalp above the opening (Berger, 1929). He took this as evidence that the EEG did not originate in the scalp. He tried to eliminate eye and other movements as a cause, both by comparing records of actual eye movements with EEG records and by making sure that subjects remained still during recordings.

In repeating his work, Adrian and Matthews (1934) found that neither passive nor active movements of the eyes produced any detectable effect on potentials recorded between the occiput and the vertex, and that the recordable effects (such as those produced by blinking) were at their greatest in the neighbourhood of the eyes, whereas the alpha rhythm was at its greatest over the occiput. They also confirmed Berger's observation in patients with trephined skulls that the alpha rhythm was greatest when one of the electrodes was over the hole and the other one over the occiput.

Further experiments by Adrian and Yamigawa (1935) confirmed alpha blocking phenomena and also showed, using a corpse, that electrodes at the scalp surface could indeed be used to pick up signals emanating from a dipole generator placed inside the brain.

In spite of the cautious attitude adopted by the early workers, there have periodically been suggestions that the alpha rhythm is artefactual, caused either by pulsations in the cortex resulting from changes in blood pressure or by movements of the eyes. One good reason for this is that is difficult to conceive how such regular sinusoidal waves could be generated by nerve cells whose own electrical activity has always been regarded as being exclusively spikey. Adrian and Matthews suggested that the alpha rhythm represented a spontaneous beat in a group of cortical neurons, that the neurons depolarised almost simultaneously and that the gross EEG represents the envelope of the activity of the underlying tissue. The gross EEG, recorded from the other side of a centimetre of bone, skin and fat, was thought to represent a blurred and averaged picture of the sum of the activity of many individual cells. An essential prediction of this model is that individual cells cannot produce a typical EEG trace, and neither can small groups of cells – their spikes would be individually represented rather than being blurred and run together into a smooth waveform.

In fact, however, recordings from small areas of cortex do not confirm this view. As early as 1936, Gerard found that wave activity persisted in small fragments of frog brain tissue. More recently, Elul (1972) implanted microelectrodes in the brains of experimental animals and found that wave-like EEG activity could be recorded when the electrodes were only 30 μm apart. Sophisticated filtering techniques ensured that 'background' activity was eliminated, and only the local fluctuations in potential between the two points were recorded: 'If the EEG is produced through summation of a large number of spike potentials, as proposed by Adrian and Matthews (1934), clearly differential recordings should become increasingly spike-like as the volume of tissue (and consequently the number of nerve cells) producing the activity is made smaller. Yet, it became evident in the study that wave activity recorded between two electrodes only 30 mu apart was as EEG-like in character as that recorded between two electrodes several centimetres apart. In fact, decreasing the inter-electrode separation had no appreciable effect on the wave activity recorded differentially between them. These results can be interpreted only as a contradiction of the Adrian–Matthews model (Elul, 1972)'.

Given that the EEG is produced in the cortex, how else could it arise than from the spike activity of nerve cells? It must be the summation of either slow graded activity of neurons or their supporting cells, the glial cells. Both have been suggested as the origin of the EEG. Galambos (1961) drew attention to the fact that glial cells outnumber neurons by ten to one in the human cortex, which gives it the highest glial index in the animal kingdom. He therefore argued for more research on glial functions, and also suggested that the glia, rather than neurons, may be responsible for brainwaves, since the similarity of EEG activity throughout the brain well reflects the uniformity in size of glia, while neurons vary enormously in size, number and arrangement, in different parts.

Elul rejects this view, pointing out that the changes in potential produced by glial cells are too slow to produce an EEG waveform. Also, drugs that specifically block the activity of neurons but leave the glial cells functioning relatively normally also block the EEG entirely. Of course, evidence like this, where the administration of a drug results in the cessation of some natural activity, should be treated with caution: it may be that the glial cells are also affected by the drug, but not as obviously as the neurons. It could still be argued that EEG may be exclusively produced by the glia in normal circumstances, or even in conjunction with neurons.

The slow changes in neuronal synaptic potential have also been offered as candidates for the origin of EEG (for instance, by Purpura, 1959). Elul discounts these potentials as well – if they did summate to produce EEG in the cortex, then there seems no logical reason why they should not do so in the spinal cord as well, which is just as densely populated with equally large excitatory and inhibitory synaptic potentials as many parts of the cortex. He suggested instead that the EEG is generated in the cell membrane, in fairly small patches, 'probably including several synapses and some passive membrane through which the synaptic current returns into the cell', and that these groups of synapses may represent functional units.

Another model of the way the human EEG, and the alpha rhythm in particular, is generated has been proposed by Andersen and Andersen (1968). Although all their experimental work has been on cats, they believe that the EEG activity of the cat, while under barbiturate anaesthesia, is sufficiently similar to the human EEG to allow conclusions to be drawn from the intracranial recordings of the activities of individual cells and cell nuclei. Essentially, they found that the activity in the cat which is apparent at the scalp is generated by the pyramidal neurons (long nerve cells) in the underlying cortex, and that they are kept in synchrony by generators in the thalamus, an area of the brain lying under the cortex, in man, in the centre of the cranium.

The origin of scalp-recorded waveforms can thus be determined, in animals, by systematic triangulation with intracranial electrodes. This is obviously not possible in man, and neurophysiologists simply do not know for certain how the human EEG is generated: the evidence from animals is as yet unconfirmed. There is, however, absolutely no doubt that electrical activity originating in the human cortex can be measured from the scalp.

ATTEMPTS TO IDENTIFY THE FOCUS OF ORIGIN OF ALPHA

On the basis of their observations of the relative independence of the waveforms from the two sides of the head, Adrian and Yamigawa (1935) proposed two foci for alpha, one in each occipital lobe. Walsh (1958) used an electronic 'wave correlator' to compare the phase relations of alpha from the two sides of the head, and came to the same conclusion.

A more sophisticated study, using a 48-channel recording system and the construction of equipotential field maps, was reported by Lehmann (1971). Three scalp areas were associated with maximal and minimal values, indicating proximity to the origin of activity in the alpha range — the left and right occiputs, and a central, parietal/vertex location. This is not necessarily contradicting the previous two findings, in that the central origin could be a reflection of the mu, or rolandic, rhythm, also running at about 10 Hz. It is odd, however, if this was so, that two generators, one over each sensorimotor cortex, were also not evident for this rhythm. A third possible explanation is that a central alpha generator exists for alpha, and it is expressed independently in the two occipital lobes. Henderson *et al.* (1976) assumed a common generator for all the alpha generated on the scalp, and derived a position from multichannel recordings, corresponding to the ventrolateral nucleus of the left thalamus, from which all the alpha activity could have originated. This corresponds with the evidence offered by Andersen and Andersen, discussed in the previous section, indicating that generators in the thalamus may be crucial in the generation of synchronous waves on the scalp.

To sum up, scalp recordings indicate that alpha activity originates deep in the centre of the brain and is expressed somewhat independently on the left and right occiputs, presumably modulated by activity in the left and right occipital lobes.

THE PHENOMENA OF THE ALPHA RHYTHM

The most obvious rhythmic activity in the EEG is at 10 Hz. In fact, to the untrained eye using unsophisticated high-inertia pen galvanometers this is the only plainly noticeable activity that can be recorded from normal awake subjects. Early workers (such as Adrian and Matthews, 1934) actually used the word 'electrencephalogram', or the term 'Berger rhythm', simply to refer to 10 Hz activity recorded from the scalp; and only when it was realised that other rhythms and patterns of electrical activity could also be detected was a special name — the 'alpha rhythm' — applied to 10 Hz activity.

Adrian and Matthews also found that alpha disappeared specifically when the scalp. It is at its greatest amplitude at the rear of the head, the occiput, and is normally only evident when the subject has closed the eyes and is relatively relaxed. The alpha rhythm disappears if the subject's attention is fully occupied — for instance, by performing mental arithmetic — and returns again as soon as the subject stops concentrating. This phenomenon is called 'alpha blocking'. It is very easily elicited. (See example in Figure 1.6.)

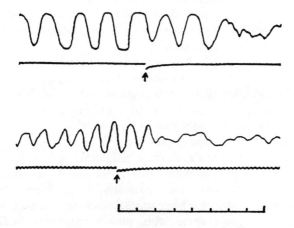

Figure 1.6 Blocking of occipital alpha rhythm by light stimulus. The upper two traces show the 5 Hz rhythm of a 1-year-old child attenuated after 0.4 s, the lower two the 10 Hz rhythm of an adult attenuated after 0.2 s. From Bernhard and Skoglund (1943)

Adrian and Matthews also found that alpha disappeared specifically when the subject focused the eyes on something: it could be produced when the eyes were open, but confronted by a uniform visual field (an arrangement of an opal glass bowl in front of the face, lit by a ring of lamps). Clearly strongly inhibited by focused visual stimulation, the alpha rhythm could also be 'driven' by a flickering light. Adrian and Matthews found that it was possible to obtain as high as 25 Hz under suitable conditions, and also that flicker at 10 Hz potentiated alpha, doubling its amplitude compared with when the eyes were closed, without stimulation.

The essential phenomena of alpha rhythm were established 50 years ago, and it can be argued that little more is known about it now. Our understanding of the physiology of EEG as a whole has also developed somewhat slowly over this period. In the next section there is an account of a very serious challenge to the accepted view that alpha originates in the brain. This proposition generated an animated debate in the academic journals during the early 1970s, strikingly illustrating how, despite forty years of research and a similarly long history of clinical application of EEG techniques, very little indeed was known of the origin or significance of the EEG's most obvious component, alpha.

MODERN EVIDENCE ON THE ORIGIN OF THE ALPHA RHYTHM

An astonishingly persuasive challenge to the accepted view that alpha arose in the occipital cortex was put forward in 1970 by Olof Lippold, whose theory about alpha being caused by eye tremor actually accounted for all the classically known facts about it. He also had experimental evidence in support of his model. No account of the significance of this pervasive rhythm would be complete without a consideration of his model, even though it turns out to have been inadequate as a complete explanation.

Lippold, a physiologist who has spent much of his research career working on muscle activity, had long been impressed by the similarity between alpha rhythm and muscular tremor. Muscle trembles at about 10 Hz when it is inactive, in an awake person. During purposive movement this tremor normally disappears, and muscle tone drops during deep relaxation or sleep to levels at which the tremor is no longer measurable. Muscle tension is determined by an efferent nerve from the spinal cord, and the nerve's activity is modulated by information coming to the spinal cord from stretch-sensitive cells in the muscle, via afferent fibres. A slight delay in this loop means that the system is very easily set into tremor. When purposive movements are being made, muscle tension is determined by a completely different, goal-oriented, set of reflexes, and the tremor disappears.

Lippold's hypothesis was essentially that when the eye is shut, the muscles controlling its movement will show tremor, just as any other muscles do, and that this tremor will result in movement of the eyeball. At the back of the eye is the light-sensitive layer of tissues known as the retina, and across this is a standing electrical potential of about a millivolt (the corneoretinal potential) — a massive charge in electrophysiological terms. (Remember that EEGs are normally calibrated in *micro*volts.) Any movement of the eye will result in a change in electrical field, especially in the front of the head. (Our normal method of measuring eye movements, using the electro-oculogram, is based on this fact.) It was Lippold's belief that somehow these changes in potential reverberate through the skull, so that they are most easily measurable at the occiput, in the EEG, where they manifest themselves as the alpha rhythm.

In order to test this hypothesis, Lippold cooled one eye while simultaneously warming the other, with water, and found that the alpha rhythm on the cooled side (measured occipitally) was slower than that on the warm side. He suggested that this was caused by a difference in the delay inherent in the stretch reflex arc for the two eyes, caused by the temperature difference. Similarly, he systematically altered the size of the corneoretinal potential by exposing subjects' eyes to different levels of illumination, and found that alpha amplitude was very closely correlated with the size of the corneoretinal potential, as his theory would predict.

Not surprisingly, Lippold's theory received a great deal of attention. An essential prediction of the model is that people without eyes (normally, who have been enucleated for clinical reasons) should show no alpha rhythm, as they have no corneoretinal potential. Generally speaking, blind people show little or no alpha rhythm. A report of an eyeless subject showing some alpha rhythm was rejected by Lippold after he had thoroughly examined this subject himself. Despite the fact that the patient had no retina (or choroid), the membrane lining the eye was in a constant state of fluttering. Lippold interpreted these facts as showing that the source of alpha was not in fact the extraocular muscles and the corneoretinal potential, but the stumps of muscle and linings of the orbit, although it was not clear how this activity could be transformed into occipital activity.

A more direct test of a peripheral explanation of the alpha rhythm was reported by Cavonius and Estevez-Uscaryn (1974), making use of a piece of apparatus which allowed of the stimulation of the left and right visual cortex separately. (The sensory nerves from the eye systematically go to either the left or right hemisphere, depending on which half of the visual field, in either eye, they came from.) They found that patterned stimulation only caused alpha blocking on one side of the head (ipsilateral to the side of the visual field that was being used, as would be predicted from anatomy), despite the fact that *both* eyes received identical information. This seemed to dispose of Lippold's theory conclusively, although the evidence about alpha correlating with the size of the corneoretinal potential remains unexplained. A later replication (Tait and Pavlovski, 1978) failed to repeat Lippold's observation of a change in alpha amplitude resulting from a change in corneoretinal potential. (This was not because the authors had failed to gain control of corneoretinal potential amplitude, as they showed that their subjects' potentials were shifted by the changes in ambient illumination at least as much as Lippold's.) Attractive and stimulating though it may be, we may therefore reject Lippold's theory quite confidently as an explanation for all the 10 Hz activity measurable at the occipital scalp. The real significance of his model is in demonstrating how little more we know about EEG and alpha rhythm than did Hans Berger in 1929, and also in pointing out the necessity for considering physiological mechanisms in the visual system when attempting to explain alpha.

Wertheim (1974) has developed a hypothesis which, like Lippold's, links alpha rhythm intimately to the control and feedback systems of the eyes. Attentive behaviour is always accompanied by the use of oculomotor feedback in normally sighted people, and Wertheim (1981) suggested that it is the use of afferent information from the retina about eye position and movement which attenuated alpha rhythm. That is, alpha is not generated peripherally but is blocked by the use of peripheral feedback from the eyes. In his own words: '. . .the degree of desynchronization of the occipital EEG is unrelated to visual information processing but can be taken to reflect the degree to which retinal information is used in oculmotor control (Wertheim, 1981)'.

Experiments in which alpha activity was assessed with a by-pass filter during the performance of a pursuit rotor task showed that it was maximal when the movements of the target were regular and predictable. When the subjects made errors under these conditions (and consequently were obliged to use retinal feedback to correct their tracking performance), alpha activity was reduced. When the target moved unpredictably, alpha activity was very low both during successful performance and following errors. Wertheim used reaction time data to show that the level of information processing was not significantly reduced during the easy task, when reaction times were at their shortest, and was apparently unrelated to the amount of alpha during stimulus presentation.

While Wertheim's work has impressively identified retinal afference as being of prime importance in determining the expression of alpha activity, and therefore supports the notion that alpha originates in the thalamus, as Andersen and Andersen had suggested, it says little about its function. Theories developed to ascribe a function to the alpha rhythm will be dealt with at the end of the next chapter. It is clear from the evidence discussed here that alpha is not entirely artefactual (although it is possible that a small proportion of 10 Hz activity is generated corneoretinally) and that its expression is determined largely by peripheral oculomotor functions.

2

The Alpha Rhythm, Other Brainwaves and States of Mind

EEG, GENETICS AND INDIVIDUAL DIFFERENCES

While it is accepted that physical characteristics such as eye colour, height or size of cranium are largely determined by heredity, it is by no means clear how genetic influences shape psychological traits — intellectual or emotional. The EEG is naturally determined by factors such as the size and shape of the cranium and idiosyncracies in anatomy of the underlying tissues, as well as by any functional characteristics of the brain. It would be unsurprising if the brainwaves characteristic of one member of a family were not shared by others, given the first set of reasons. Whether this similarity reflects functional similarities in the ways in which their brains work — their psychological traits — is a different matter, depending on the heritability of those traits and the degree to which they contribute to EEG variability.

Genetic (Twin) Studies

Identical (monozygotic) twins produce very similar EEG patterns. Vogel (1970) reported on a series of studies of 208 twins, 110 of whom were monozygotic, claiming that it was possible for a scorer to identify one twin's EEG from the other's, blind, for monozygotic pairs, although not for dizygotic. The age of the subjects seemed unimportant, which indicates the degree of stability of EEG characeristics. Similarly, spectral analysis of twins, EEGs by Clarke and Harding (1969) showed an advantage over visual inspection in discriminating the greater similarity between 10 monozygotic pairs than between 10 dizygotics.

Using visual evoked potentials, Dustman and Beck (1965) correlated the averaged signals between monozygotic twins, dizygotic twins and unrelated children, showing that the latter two groups had similar degrees of concordance (r approximately +0.6), while the identical pairs' correlations varied between

+0.7 and +0.8, depending on electrode placement. There is therefore very good evidence that heredity plays a large part in determining both spontaneous and event-related EEG characteristics. Of course, whether this has any functional significance is a different matter.

EEG and Psychological Traits

One of Berger's hopes for the EEG was that it would contribute to psychiatry in permitting the diagnosis of types of psychiatric illness as well as reflecting variations in personality. With the exception of its application in the diagnosis of epilepsy, it was established very soon that the EEG could not discriminate patients according to their psychiatric diagnosis. However, there have been continuing attempts to correlate EEG indices with psychological traits, including psychopathy, extraversion, facility with visual imagery, creativity and general intelligence.

A major problem with this enterprise is illustrated very well by the research into 'imagery types' and alpha rhythm. Golla *et al*. (1943) classified people into groups depending on whether they reported being able to visualise or not, and also into EEG categories of persistent alpha types (people producing alpha with eyes open or closed), responsive types (the 'normals', showing alpha with eyes closed, but not when they were open) and minus types (who never showed any alpha during the experiment). They found a very encouragingly large preponderance of visualisers in the alpha-minus category and of non-visualisers in the persistent alpha category. One problem with this experiment lies in its classification according to EEG criteria: Oswald (1957) showed quite clearly that very few people indeed produce no alpha, and the so-called alpha-minus types will produce alpha rhythm if given the chance — allowed to relax, to settle down properly, and so on. Thus, in his experiment the visualisers, given the opportunity, showed almost as much evidence of alpha rhythm (of the responsive sort) as the non-visualisers in some other experiments. That is, the amount of alpha rhythm in EEG is not entirely an enduring characteristic of the individual, but reflects the outcome of the interaction between the individual and the experimental situation and its consequence for their level of cortical activity. The close relationship between alpha activity and the functioning of the visual system was discussed at greater length in Chapter 1. In particular, the work of Wertheim (1974, 1981), suggesting that alpha amplitude is determined by the degree to which retinal information is used in oculomotor control, could be used to explain any correlation of EEG with differences in cognitive style, particularly when it involves differences in habits of visualisation.

Because the alpha rhythm is an involuntary response, which the subject is not even aware of, it is tempting to equate it with innately determined characteristics such as sleep mechanisms. Linking cognitive styles to alpha-responsiveness then appears to say something about the origin and stability of the former. It would be more accurate to state the relationship between alpha and cognition by saying that, whereas individuals may have habitual strategies of thinking, mirrored in their EEG, it does not mean to say that they are unable, by changing their mental strategy, to change their EEG.

Alpha amplitude is widely recognised as a good measure of cortical arousal (see next section). A major interpretation of the origin of differences in extraversion — Eysenck's (1967) theory — is that extroverts and introverts innately exhibit a level of arousal which is below or above the optimal level. The theory ascribes all the differences attributable to this trait, including sociability and impulsiveness, to this essential neurophysiological difference between introverts and extroverts. Under the same conditions, therefore, extroverts, being less aroused, should show a less activated EEG, with more alpha rhythm, than introverts. Gale (1973) reviewed the relevant studies since 1938, observing no consensus in their findings and thus little support for this simple model. Rather than abandoning the theory, however, Gale argues that adaptive strategies normally adopted by extroverts and introverts specifically relate to manipulating arousal level, and that, in any case, no simple difference ought to be expected. As in the correlation of running EEG measures with imagery type, it is clear that situational factors are overwhelmingly important. In the case of extraversion, the variable one is trying to measure (personality) positively interacts with the situation, especially if it is very boring, as EEG experiments often are!

A most promising development has been the correlation of some aspects of the auditory evoked potential (AEP) with measures of intelligence. Ertl and Schafer (1969) reported differences in latency of some AEP components in subjects of very low intelligence compared with normals — the brighter subjects showing faster EEG responses. Using 100 subjects representing the full range of IQ, Shucard and Horn (1973) confirmed this finding with a very low (although statistically significant) correlation in the same direction. To put it simply, the faster a brain works the more intelligent the individual will be, and the shorter the latency of evoked potentials to simple stimuli. This work was followed up by Blinkhorn and Hendrickson (1982), who had what they claimed to be an even better EEG measure of intelligence. Using 33 subjects, they showed that IQ — assessed by the Ravens Progressive Matrices — correlated positively with what they called a 'string' measure of the AEP. This measure is an estimate of the complexity of the waveform produced — as though the average were stretched out like a piece of string. The size of their correlations (from 0.5 to 0.75) is of the same order of magnitude as correlations between the subtests of an intelligence test. If reliable, this would be a most significant advance, not only in our understanding of the nature of intelligence, but also as providing a straightforward, culture-free method of estimating intelligence level. This finding remains highly controversial. The relatively small size of the samples involved (as far as correlational work goes) and the continuing lack of any confirmation of their two reports does not inspire confidence.

EEG AS A REFLECTION OF ALERTNESS

Arousal theory involves the idea of a continuum of nervous activation ranging from deep sleep to high emotional excitement, and was first formulated by Duffy (1934). This notion was important in treating the nervous system as more than simply a mechanism for responding to environmental demands. It proposed that emotional and motivational forces give rise to resultant levels of activation or arousal which remain somewhat independent of stimulus events. Neuro-physiologists — notably Bremer and Lindsley — working on the isolated cortex preparation were able to show that the nervous system did not lapse into inactivity when all stimulation was denied. Moruzzi and Magoun (1949) finally identified the reticular activation system as the mechanism that satisfied the requirements of Duffy's theory in that its activity could be demonstrated to maintain the cortex at a level of excitation not always dependent on stimulation. In addition, other hindbrain structures were shown to be largely responsible for sleep. These breakthroughs in physiology gave spectacular credence to arousal theory, which was taken up enthusiastically by psychologists such as Lindsley (1951), Hebb (1955) and Malmo (1959). The establishment of psychological theory in physio-logical discovery received its most significant boost this century with this con-firmation with neurophysiological evidence of a previously entirely psychological model.

    Although arousal is useful as an explanatory concept and well founded in neurophysiology, no single psychophysiological measure of arousal has emerged. While parameters sensitive to autonomic changes — e.g. galvanic skin response, finger pulse volume or heart rate — normally covary (see, e.g., Hassett, 1978), this is not invariably the case. There are a number of possible reasons for this, which are beyond the scope of this chapter, but, in any case, measures of auto-nomic activity are a very indirect estimate of cortical activation. Techniques that have been assessed as more direct measures of cortical arousal include EEG, critical flicker fusion, sedation threshold and even the persistence of the spiral after-effect. Gross changes in state, such as deep sleep to awake alertness, are, of course, reflected in easily detected EEG changes. The EEG is also an excellent measure of depth of sleep. Lindsley (1952) articulated the relationship between EEG measures, levels of awareness and behavioural efficiency in a way that has become widely accepted and experimentally very useful (see Table 2.1).

    On-line frequency analysis can be used to assess power of different wavebands, such as alpha and theta, and this sort of measurement can be particularly useful at low levels of arousal, from light sleep upwards.

Effects of Sleep Deprivation

Sleep deprivation results in measurable decreases in alpha activity in resting adults, indicating a lowered level of arousal. Williams *et al.* (1959), who first reported this, also found that errors perpetrated during a vigilance task were

Table 2.1 Psychological states and their EEG, conscious and behavioural correlates (after Lindsley, 1952)

Behavioural continuum	Electro-encephalogram	State of awareness	Behavioural efficiency
Strong, excited emotion (fear, rage, anxiety)	Desynchronised; low to moderate amplitude; fast mixed	Restricted awareness; divided attention	Poor (lack of control, freezing-up, disorganised)
Alert attentiveness	Partially synchronised: mainly fast, low-amplitude waves	Selective attention, but may vary or shift. 'Concentration'	Good (efficient, selective, quick, reactions)
Relaxed wakefulness	Synchronised: optimal alpha rhythm	Attention wanders — not forced. Favours free association	Good (routine reactions and creative thought)
Drowsiness	Reduced alpha and occasional low-amplitude slow waves	Borderline, partial awareness. Imagery and reverie	Poor (unco-ordinated, sporadic, lacking timing)
Light sleep	Spindle bursts and slow waves. Loss of alpha	Markedly reduced consciousness (loss of consciousness). Dream state	Absent
Deep sleep	Large and very slow waves (synchrony but on slow time base)	Complete loss of awareness (no memory for stimulation or for dreams)	Absent
Coma	Isoelectric to irregular large waves	Complete loss of consciousness; little or no response to stimulation. Amnesia	Absent
Death	Isoelectric: gradual and permanent loss of EEG activity	Complete loss of awareness as death ensues	Absent

associated with particularly low levels of alpha activity in these subjects, which suggested that they were periodically slipping into even lower levels of arousal. Naitoh and Townsend (1970) confirmed that the lapses occurring in monotonous counting and adding tasks in sleep-deprived subjects were associated with low alpha activity, and, in fact, all the EEG characteristics of light sleep. This sort of finding has been taken as support for the 'lapse theory' of the effects of sleep loss − that sleepy people can perform just as well as normally with the exertion of some effort but that they suffer from periodic lapses of attention or action caused by a sudden lowering of arousal, perhaps even resulting in a microsleep.

Both behavioural and EEG evidence is available to support lapse theory as an explanation of the decrements in performance following sleep loss. A more important theoretical point, relevant to the dynamics of arousal mechanisms and ultimately to the functions of sleep itself, concerns whether this is the *only* difference between a sleepy person and a rested one. Event-related potential studies (e.g. Naitoh *et al.*, 1969, 1971, 1973) show changes in EEG with sleep deprivation, but, of course, they inevitably confound trials on which subjects may have been responding normally with trials on which they were inattentive or inactive.

Recent behavioural evidence (Lisper and Kjellberg, 1972; Tharp, 1978) suggests that the 'normal' fast responding of the sleep-deprived subject is actually slower than normal. Inspection of the data presented by Williams *et al.* (1959) in their seminal monograph clearly shows that their subjects were also performing less well when sleep-deprived, even on their fast, 'normal' trials.

Ideally, we would like to be able to compare the EEG during periods of so-called normal responding with EEG during lapses, when responses are unusually slow or non-existent. A graduate student in Hull has attempted to do just this, using the contingent negative variation (Lister, 1981). In this experimental paradigm a warning stimulus (S1) is followed after a brief interval (the inter-stimulus interval, or ISI) by an imperative stimulus (S2) to which a simple response is required. Negativity developing centrally on the scalp is the CNV, or expectancy wave.

Since a response is invariably involved in recording the CNV, it is possible to separate the CNV recordings preceding fast, 'normal' responses from those preceding the ultra-slow responses associated with lapses. Taking the 8 fastest and 8 slowest trials out of a total of 56, Lister found, like Lisper and Kjellberg, that although slow trials were disproportionately slower after sleep loss (over 20 per cent), the fast trials after sleep loss were 10 per cent slower as well. After normal sleep the CNVs associated with fast responses were greater than those associated with slow responses. (This is in line with most of the available evidence on rested subjects − see Papakostopoulos and Fenelon, 1975.) However, after sleep loss this relationship was reversed − fast responses were associated with very-low-amplitude CNVs. In another experiment Lister showed that anticipatory CNVs in a 30 min vigilance task steadily declined in amplitude over time after sleep loss, but gradually increased in amplitude in the rested subject. The effects of sleep loss therefore seem to be in reducing the alerting properties of stimulation, and CNV amplitude seems to mirror closely this decline in recruitment of arousal, which has to increase steadily during the 30 min in the rested subject, in this intrinsically boring de-arousing task.

The application of EEG techniques has increased our understanding of the behavioural effects of sleep loss, confirming the existence of lapses as symptoms of failures of arousal. It has also been crucial in the development of theory about the significance of these lapses, and in showing that lapses are not the only symptoms of sleepiness — the sleep-deprived subject is slower, and has different EEG even when performing at his or her best.

Drug Effects

The drugs which affect behaviour — psychotropic drugs — can all be categorised as being cortical depressants or cortical stimulants. The former include the barbiturates, tranquillisers, cannabis and alcohol; the latter, caffeine and the amphetamines. In the same way that alcohol and tranquillisers may both act as cortical depressants, yet have very different effects on behaviour and mood, so the effects of drugs on EEG are predictable in terms of their effects on arousal, and yet also have signatures of their own. In this way the barbiturates, for instance, produce an EEG typical of low activation in a co-operative subject, but also typically produce beta activity (14–30 Hz), increasingly so as the dose increases to become sedative. Sedative doses of diazepam or other benzodiazepines (minor tranquillisers) also produce abundant beta.

Doses of cannabis or alcohol consistent with recreational usage have no such peculiar effects, the EEG reflecting merely the level of arousal resulting from the interaction of drug effects on the individual (see e.g., Koukkou and Lehmann, 1976). Thus, the drowsy hallucinations of cannabis intoxication (similar in many ways to some peoples' normal hypnagogic imagery) are associated with reduced alpha and increased theta, while the relatively alert drugged individual produces a relatively 'normal' EEG.

The EEG during deep anaesthesia or drug overdose is totally different from the normal picture, an outcome of the brain in acute distress, and is characterised by bursts of slow waves separated by periods of almost complete electrical silence. Binnie *et al.* (1982) suggest that this pattern indicates the relative isolation of the cortex from the underlying white matter, presumably as a result of a differential uptake of the drug by different tissues.

This section started with the assertion that the physiological underpinning of the concept of arousal was one of the most important points of interaction between psychology and physiology this century. It must be clear by now that although undoubtedly useful in explaining behaviour, the arousal concept itself remains somewhat ill-expressed in terms of measurable psychological phenomena. The EEG is probably the best psychophysiological technique for estimating arousal and its relation to attention and effort.

HYPNOSIS, MEDITATION AND TRANCE STATES

Hypnosis

Sleeping brainwaves were successfully distinguished from waking ones by the Loomis group during the 1930s, and a full account of their work is given in Chapter 5. This advance encouraged them to try to distinguish other states of consciousness such as hypnosis. Early attempts (see, e.g., Loomis *et al.*, 1936) proved disappointing, showing no difference in EEG during hypnotic trance compared with normal wakefulness. There followed a number of reports of similarity between the EEG during hypnosis and light sleep or drowsiness (Barker and Burgwin, 1949; Israel and Rohmer, 1958; Chertok and Kramarz, 1959).

Before we become deeply involved in the methodological issues that may account for these equivocal findings, it may be useful to consider the evidence for hypnosis being different from wakefulness, in any case. Recent sceptics such as Barber (1969) have questioned the whole idea that hypnosis results in a state of trance, arguing that a large element of role-playing is involved for most people being hypnotised. Many apparently 'good' hypnotic subjects will admit, if it is suggested to them, that they are unsure themselves whether they 'really' become hypnotised or are only pretending. What is certain is that hypnotic susceptibility is a relatively stable trait and that it can be measured by standard questionnaires. Studies comparing the EEG of highly susceptible with hypnotically non-susceptible subjects have provided some interesting results.

Galbraith *et al.* (1970) set out to determine the best EEG determinants of scores on the Harvard Group Susceptibility Scale, from a variety of EEG measures. This multivariate approach showed that four of the five best predictors of susceptibility were in the theta range, and the best one was the 5 Hz component of vertex EEG, recorded with the eyes open. Tebecis *et al.* (1975) compared a group of practised self-hypnotists with normal controls, also finding that theta activity was greater in hypnotically adept subjects.

The maintenance of a hypnotic trance, whether the outcome of role-playing or not, essentially involves the control and focusing of attention. It has been suggested that theta activity may reflect some aspects of attentional processes (Schachter, 1977), and these results are consistent with that view; but, as Schachter points out himself, they are also consistent with the explanation that subjects trained in relaxation (as hypnotic subjects are) or susceptible to hypnosis may relax more effectively than controls during the testing sessions, and that their theta waves may reflect the onset of drowsiness rather than any components specific to trance states. This explanation also accounts for the discrepancy between the findings mentioned at the beginning of this section, with some experimenters finding no differences between the EEG of hypnosis and normal wakefulness, and others finding evidence of sleeping EEG. Their subjects really were asleep!

Meditation

Most psychophysiological studies of meditation have used subjects practised in 'transcendental meditation' (TM). This technique was developed by Maharishi Mahesh Yogi, the guru first made famous by the Beatles, and is systematically taught and proselytised as a way of life by his organisation. Practitioners have two daily sessions of meditation, about 15–20 min each, during which they sit quietly, sometimes in a fairly uncomfortable posture. Early in their training a sound or word is given to them as their personal mantra by the teacher, and they are instructed to bring it to mind continuously during meditation, neither contemplating its meaning nor concentrating on it, but experiencing it freely and repetitively.

Objective measures of the psychophysiology of meditating subjects have given some support to the notion that there is a distinct state which is normally only achieved during meditation. Wallace and Benson (1972), for instance, reported rapid changes in a number of physiological parameters with the onset of meditation. Oxygen consumption dropped, and so did the production of carbon dioxide, which indicates a lowering of metabolic rate. There was a rapid rise in the electrical resistance of the skin and a decline in the concentration of blood lactate (both indicating a lowering in level of arousal).

Benson (1976) has extended the early work on metabolic changes, showing that subjects who had merely been instructed in relaxation methods based on meditative techniques (without any practice or the benefit of religious hocus-pocus) were able to decrease their oxygen consumption significantly more than by simply sitting with their eyes closed. Benson argues that the physiological phenomena accompanying meditation are part of what he calls the 'relaxation response', which is, he says, as naturally embedded in our nervous systems as the startle reaction. He now campaigns for periodic relaxation as a way of reducing the effects of stress, while Wallace has joined the TM establishment and is Principal of the Maharishi International University (MIU). Much of the debate about the effects of meditation and its possible benefits has been clouded by assessments of the worldly Maharishi's organisation and its methods. Nevertheless, a number of studies have been carried out evaluating meditation in its own right.

Anand *et al.* (1961) reported that the EEG of meditators showed a slowed alpha rhythm, of high amplitude, which gradually spread from the occipital to the frontal areas. Banquet (1973) confirmed the preponderance of alpha activity during meditation, but also claimed that second and third stages of meditation could be attained by more adept practitioners, in which theta frequencies ('different from those of sleep') suffused from frontal to posterior channels, appearing in short trains. Finally, and only in the most advanced subjects, came a period of very deep meditation, in which beta waves of 20–50 Hz predominated over the whole scalp. Banquet also claimed that during meditation alpha blocking did not occur to low-intensity clicks and flashes, but click stimulation did block the trains of theta activity when they occurred. These two papers are frequently quoted (especially in literature from MIU) as evidence for TM being a unique state of consciousness.

Some other experimenters have disagreed with this conclusion, that meditation represents a unique physiological state, maintaining instead that the EEG and other psychophysiological evidence is consistent with meditation being a state of light sleep. Younger's group, in fact, reported that some of their subjects developed very large slow waves in EEG typical of deep sleep (Younger *et al.*, 1975). They suggest that many of the physiological changes previously reported may have been due to unrecognised sleep activity. Most meditative techniques, including TM, involve some sort of stereotyped posture (kneeling, squatting or sitting) which is incompatible with normal sleep. The classical position for Eastern meditation is the mudra or lotus position, with the left sole on the inside of the right thigh, and vice versa. Younger's subjects were instructed to lie down during their periods of meditation in the laboratory, and it may be this that resulted in their dropping off to sleep. A more carefully controlled experiment by Fenwick's group allowed subjects to sit up in their normal way while meditating. Fenwick *et al.* (1977) confirmed Banquet's findings of increased alpha rhythm and of developing trains of theta activity, but interpreted these data as indicating that the meditator was balancing in a state of light drowsiness. They offered as evidence the fact that almost all of their subjects showed rolling eye movements during meditation, which are typical of light sleep.

EEG evidence, therefore, does not indicate anything sufficiently remarkable about meditation to merit calling it a discrete psychophysiological state. Some of the justification for doing so (in the original Wallace and Benson argument) lay in the claim that metabolic rate fell to very low 'hypometabolic' levels during meditation. In assessing changes in metabolic rate with meditation, Fenwick's group ensured that their subjects had settled down and were normally relaxed during the 'baseline' recordings. The careful establishment of the resting metabolic level is obviously crucial, if comparisons are to be made to establish whether meditation itself is hypometabolic. Fenwick's group found that the drop in oxygen consumption reported by Wallace and Benson did not occur if the initial level had been allowed to settle down properly, and concluded that the metabolic change occurring during meditation is 'related to the initial metabolic level of the subject, and the degree of subjective tension which the subjects are experiencing'. It seems that the early experiments overestimated the reduction in metabolic rate during meditation.

EEG work carried out in Hull (Barwood *et al.*, 1978) investigated the auditory evoked potential (AEP) responses of meditators to quiet click stimulation. Since meditators report that they simultaneously become sensitised to small sounds but are capable of totally ignoring them, it was predicted that we should find changes in the late components of the AEP compared with baseline. In the event, no consistent changes were found, although the evoked potentials of meditation were more similar to those of wakefulness than those of sleep. Interestingly, our subjects showed significantly fewer saccadic eye movements and blinks during meditation than during baseline periods, and did not develop any slow rolling eye movements. This pattern, of low-voltage EEG with motionless eyes, is typical of drowsiness rather than of light sleep. Not one of our eight practised meditators reported any difficulty in meditating satisfactorily caused by the periodic clicks, and the EEG evidence is consistent with the hypothesis that they were kept at a lighter level of drowsiness than Fenwick's subjects, who were allowed to meditate in silence.

It seems clear that the experience of meditation is not dependent on any specific brainwave pattern, or drowsiness, but does require the constant maintenance of a fairly low level of arousal which allows of the sort of dissociated, free-associative thinking that meditation entails.

ALPHA BIOFEEDBACK

As described in the previous section, it has long been established (since the early 1960s) that during meditation the alpha rhythm amplitude tends to increase. At that time meditation was a practice adopted by very few Westerners, and training in meditative techniques seemed difficult, if not arduous. One solution has been the simplification of meditative techniques into 'transcendental meditation', and further into the relaxation response technique proposed by Benson.

Another solution was the idea of training people to produce alpha rhythm using biofeedback techniques, reaping the benefits of meditation without the years of training. Support was offered this approach by Joe Kamiya's pioneering experiment in 1962 (Kamiya, 1967), in which subjects were required to guess whether or not they were in alpha whenever given a signal. After each guess they were given the correct answer. From being correct 50 per cent of the time on the first day, the first subject was right 65 per cent of the time on day two and 85 per cent of the time on day three, and on day five guessed correctly on every one of 400 trials. Of another 11 subjects, 8 more also showed good evidence of training in discriminating their own EEG, although none became as good as the first subject. When asked about their experience when producing alpha, the subjects reported feelings of 'not thinking'. 'letting the mind wander' or 'feeling the heart beat', while reporting visual imagery accompanying non-alpha states.

Many experimenters have subsequently confirmed that it is indeed possible to train subjects to discriminate when they are producing alpha activity, and to produce alpha EEG on demand and stop it on demand (see, e.g., Brown, 1970). Does this mean, then, that meditation has been successfully mechanised? The relationship between the conscious control of alpha and the achievement of the 'alpha experience' has been the source of some controversy. Claims that technologically given feedback can show people the possibilities of meditation or that there is a formal equivalence of the tasks of the Yogi and of the biofeedback trainee do seem to have been overly optimistic.

Beatty (1972) assessed the relative advantages of EEG alpha rhythm biofeedback and simple instructions in relaxation, both on increasing alpha production and on increasing the incidence of subjective reports of feelings of calmness. He found that the instructions in relaxation methods actually elevated alpha rhythm slightly more than biofeedback and that similar self-reported levels of low arousal were achieved with both methods. Plotkin and Cohen (Plotkin, 1976a, b; Plotkin and Cohen, 1977) have investigated the whole question of the alpha experience very critically, pointing out that although alpha rhythm may be produced during meditation, training in alpha production is no guarantee of 'karma'. In fact, alpha is normally produced by people whenever they close their eyes and are reasonably relaxed. Their experimental evidence, like Beatty's, shows no great advantage for biofeedback training over relaxation, in producing either alpha or feelings of calmness.

Alpha biofeedback is therefore no more effective than relaxation instruction in inducing the relaxation response, even when carried out in well-equipped laboratories. The simple one-channel biofeedback machines that have been marketed to help people produce either alpha or theta EEG activity can only be less effective. One individual who trained himself on a gadget designed to produce alpha rhythm happened to find himself acting as a subject in a proper EEG laboratory, when his 'alpha' was discovered to be a series of spikes at about 10 Hz: no help in relaxation and probably distinctly unhealthy (Peper, 1974). The mechanisation of consciousness must still be regarded as science fiction.

ALPHA AND TIMING MECHANISMS

Over the past 40 years speculation about the psychological significance of the alpha rhythm has repeatedly returned to the ideas of scanning, modulations in perceptual thresholds or motor preparedness. These notions fall broadly into theories about perceptual scanning mechanisms (see, e.g., Pitts and McCulloch, 1947) and variations in cortical excitability (see, e.g., Lindsley, 1952). Scanning theory treats visual perceptual processes as being similar to TV scanning mechanisms, with the alpha rhythm being produced when blank projection areas are being swept. Perceptual input is represented by a desynchronisation of this simple pattern. It seems that theories of perception have moved on from this sort of model; and while this theory has not been disproved, it no longer receives very much attention.

The idea that alpha is an indication of variations in cortical excitability or of some sort of perceptual gating has received some support, and continues to generate testable hypotheses. An obvious difficulty with this theory is that alpha is not always present, and that some subjects (about 5 per cent of the total population) never show any evidence of it at all. We could assume that the measurable activity at 10 Hz is merely epiphenomenal and that it happens to coincide with the timing of gating, or cortical excitability. The theory is considerably weakened by this. An alternative view is that alpha always reflects variation in cortical excitability — the functional significance of this arrangement is that at periods of low cortical arousal (when alpha usually becomes evident) oscillations in arousal allow of periodic sampling from the environment and the maintenance of vigilance.

Alpha Rhythm Frequency and Reaction Time

If alpha reflects some timing mechanism, then we should expect variations in alpha frequency to be reflected in variations in reaction time (RT). Surwillo (1971) has evidence that there is a good correlation between reaction time and alpha frequency (−0.81 in an early report), his subjects ranging in age from very young to very old. Could the differences in alpha frequency be the cause of the differences in reaction time? Boddy (1971) failed to find this relationship between alpha period and RT in a group that was fairly homologous with respect to age. A second experiment by Surwillo (1975) compared young (aged 3.8–17.3 years) peoples' RTs and dominant alpha frequency, confirming the direction of the relationship, although the differences in EEG period accounted for only 9 per cent of the total variance in RT associated with age. A simple causal relationship must be ruled out. A revised model offered by Surwillo (1975) holds that slower alpha signifies slower information processing rates, but shorter-duration waves only result in faster processing if the refractory time of the perceptual process involved is short. That is, alpha gating allows of 'windows' of perception at twice the alpha rate, and it is possible to 'miss' these windows through being unprepared or because a previous signal has made the perceptual channel temporarily unresponsive. Surwillo's RT evidence for this model can only be described as suggestive, equivocal as it is, and also suffering from the problem intrinsic to all RT experiments in this context, of confounding perceptual with motor components.

Another approach to this issue has been to try and train people to alter their alpha frequency and then to test their reaction times. Woodruff (1975) trained ten old (70-year-old) and ten young (24-year-old) subjects to increase or decrease their alpha frequency, using biofeedback techniques. Old and young did equally well at increasing or decreasing their alpha rhythm, although the mean changes achieved were fairly small, overall. However, by selecting responses from each subject, during periods when their EEGs were most closely approximating a criterion of 2 Hz above or below their own modal alpha frequency, Woodruff showed that responses were slower during periods of very slow alpha than during periods of very fast alpha. Interestingly enough, this was only true of trials in which biofeedback contingencies were being enforced: the reaction times collected during spontaneously occurring periods of fast or slow alpha showed no significant differences from one another. As Woodruff suggests herself, the data do not provide unequivocal support for an excitability cycle hypothesis, and it is possible that shifts in tonic level of arousal could account for the relationship between controlled EEG activity and reaction time.

Alpha Rhythm Phase and Reaction Time

A very direct test of the idea that the alpha rhythm reflects a fluctuation in excitability is to present stimuli at different phases of the rhythm and measure RT. It is by now very well documented that reaction times at different phases of alpha do differ significantly, although it is not possible to predict, with an unfamiliar subject, which phase of the rhythm initiates the fastest responses. The initial reports, by Lansing in 1957, were limited to using 8 out of 100 subjects who had sufficiently persistent alpha to allow of a fairly straightforward visual analysis of the relationship between EEG alpha phase, stimulus onset and RT. Improvements in technique have allowed a greater proportion of subjects to be used in these experiments (Callaway et al, 1962; Dustman and Beck, 1965). However, the differences in RT obtained are small (a few milliseconds) and the effects are only obtained with visual stimuli: auditory stimuli are said to be ineffective.

It has long been known that stimulus intensity is systematically related to reaction time, with more intense stimuli eliciting faster reactions. Could it be that the apparent brightness of the stimuli was greater at certain alpha phases than others? Nunn and Osselton (1974) argued, not unreasonably, that results from reaction time experiments could never be offered as conclusive evidence for perceptual shuttering theories, since they inevitably confounded perceptual with response processes — that is, changes in RT with alpha could be the result of variation on the motor as much as on the perceptual side.

Nunn and Osselton's experiment was subtle. Very brief presentations of the word 'danger' were immediately followed by a bright flash, which could be expected to partially or wholly obliterate perception of the stimulus. The measure of perception of the stimulus was the galvanic skin response (GSR). The time relation of the stimulus to the phase of any discernible alpha rhythm was noted by an independent observer, and the results showed that GSR responses (indicating an emotional response to the word 'danger') were significantly more likely to occur when the stimuli had been presented during descending and trough phases rather than during ascending and peak phases.

Persuasive though the Nunn and Osselton results are, it would still be preferable to be able to assess thresholds at different phases of alpha rather than rely on GSR measures and *post hoc* allocations of stimulus events in terms of alpha phase. Ideally, we should decide in advance whether a stimulus should be presented on the ascending or descending phase, as this would allow of the normal determination of threshold by the systematic presentation of series of stimuli increasing and decreasing in amplitude. Jorge da Silva, a postgraduate student in Hull, has written a computer program in assembly code which operates fast enough to do just that. It detects trains of alpha rhythm, and then predicts when the next peak or trough ought to occur so as to present a signal at the appropriate moment. Preliminary experiments on auditory thresholds are promising — the procedure is effective in presenting brief signals at the right times, and it seems that thresholds during ascending alpha phases are lower than during descending phases of alpha.

3

Event-related Potentials

INTRODUCTION

In a rousing Presidential address to the Society for Psychophysiological Research
in 1981, Emmanuel Donchin set out the reasons why event-related potentials
(ERPs) are of interest to psychologists. It is no longer sufficient, he said, to
demonstrate that an EEG component is a correlate of some psychological process. To be blunt, we are already aware that psychological processes are mediated
by brain events, accompanied by electrical phenomena. The exercise only
becomes worth while if the EEG techniques (initially gained, to be sure, by the
analysis of components and correlates) can be used to throw new light on the
psychological processes themselves.

What follows is by no means an attempt at a definitive review of all the work
which has been done, which would require a book to itself. It is instead a selection
of what seem to be the most important or exemplary findings, with summaries
of the current state of knowledge assessed in relation to the considerable ambition
articulated by Donchin. This chapter provides evidence to show that this ambition not only is achievable in principle with the techniques available, but also
has already been attained in one or two instances. Excellent detailed reviews of
each of the sections dealt with are also available, and are referred to in the text.

ANALYSIS BY COMPONENT

To recapitulate some of the material in Chapter 1, event-related potentials are
assessed by averaging the EEGs associated with a number of stimulus presentations or other external events. Conventionally, the peaks and troughs in the
averaged waveform are labelled 'P' or 'N', depending on whether they were
positive or negative, the P or N being followed by a number indicating the
latency in milliseconds from the stimulus (see Figure 3.1). However, the most
well-established components are normally labelled 'N1', 'P2' and 'N2', in order

to cope with the large variations in latency which they show — for instance, with modality of stimulus.

As was indicated in Chapter 1, an essential assumption of averaging EEG waveforms is that few if any habituation or practice effects occur. In this way a large number of individual EEG responses may be used, with the effect of 'averaging out' EEG activity unrelated to the stimulus — treating this activity as being randomly varying with respect to the stimulus.

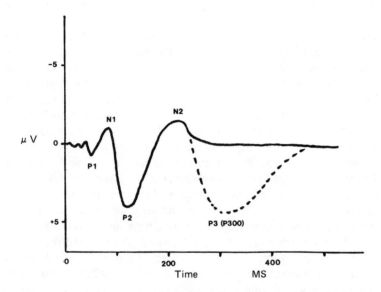

Figure 3.1 An idealised event-related potential, showing the major components between 40 and 500 ms

The first EEG responses recordable from the scalp occur too soon after the stimulus to have travelled from the sensory organ involved to the cortex. The first 25 ms of evoked potentials (EPs) are called 'far-field' recordings for this reason — they could only originate in the hindbrain, as it takes longer than 20 ms for action potentials to reach the cortex from the eye or the ear. These evoked potentials have also been labelled 'exogenous', as they are determined entirely by the physical parameters of the stimulus — they are evidence of neurological response, but not in any sense of evaluation. It would be reasonable to assume that they do not habituate. By analogy, one can also label later components of the evoked potential exogenous if they seem unresponsive to psychological variables but dependent on stimulus parameters. Exogenous components are unlikely candidates to be correlates of the sorts of psychological functions which Donchin was referring to in his Presidential address.

Later components of event-related potentials are labelled 'endogenous', which indicates that their size and latency are determined by psychological variables rather than physical parameters. Regan (1972) makes the useful distinction between experiments in which the subject is *responding to* a stimulus and those in which he or she is *evaluating* the stimulus, and it would not be surprising to find that habituation and other practice effects are more important in the latter than in the former types of experiment. We know from experiments on frog's leg and squid axon preparations that habituation effects are not intrinsic to peripheral nervous tissue (not surprisingly) — these nerve cells respond the same way whenever they are stimulated, within the limits of exhaustion or overstimulation and resulting tetanus.

Direct evidence on the origin of event-related components and their lability requires the implantation of electrodes in the human brain, and rarely is this called for clinically. One of the few reports giving this sort of evidence was by Grey Walter in 1964. He found that responses to light stimuli from within the visual cortex were dependent on the physical properties of the stimuli and did not habituate (conforming to the criteria for exogenous components). Responses from elsewhere in the cortex depended on other factors, such as alertness, and did habituate (as one would expect of endogenous components.) However, there was no clear temporal separation of these elements. In fact, both early and late components could originate in both primary and non-primary cortex.

The neuroanatomical evidence, therefore, indicates that activity before a certain interval after a stimulus cannot automatically be classified as being exogenous and all activity after that as endogenous. In addition, the late components which do reflect complex psychological processes will show practice effects such as habituation, as well as varying as a result of purely subjective determinants, such as anticipation. Using very few (up to 20) sweeps avoids this problem to some extent, and this practice is usually adopted with slow waves such as the contingent negative variation (CNV), where the signal/noise ratio of the components being assessed is large enough to average out background activity in a few sweeps. Another approach is to keep all the EEG responses and use principal components analysis (PCA) to extract evoked potential components as well as taking averages, and to use one method to confirm the results of the other. Components such as processing negativity, mismatch negativity and the P300 have relatively low signal/noise ratios with respect to the background EEG activity, so that a large number of sweeps is essential to their detection, and very careful attention has to be paid to the timing and predictability of stimuli which will affect subjects' anticipation of events. (This issue, of particular importance to the components associated with attentional processes, will be developed later.) PCA has been used in this context to investigate component structure, although the application of this technique is laborious and the outcome has so far usually been disappointingly inconclusive.

The identification of new components has always been done by the trained eye, and it is of considerable interest whether this is as reliable an instrument as its owner would normally assume. Kramer (1985) tested the accuracy and reliability of judgement of ten experienced ERP workers, using computer-generated pairs of waveforms for them to assess in terms of similarity, and assessed their performance by use of a multidimensional scaling procedure. The observers were capable of recovering the underlying dimensions of the simulated ERPs, and showed good evidence of consistency in the importance they attached to different aspects of the waveforms. As Kramer concluded, judgement of ERPs based on visual inspection can be both accurate and reliable.

EARLY COMPONENTS

Conventionally, all EEG activity averaged in about the first 80 ms is regarded as being exogenous, as it is unresponsive to psychological variables, such as evaluation of the stimulus, decision-making or any linguistic processing. Some later components (e.g. in response to visual stimulation) share these properties. Unsurprisingly, these potentials are highly specific to the modality involved, as there are, of course, great differences in the transducing mechanisms and sub-cortical neural pathways between the senses.

Auditory evoked potential (AEP) far-field brainstem potentials can be recorded during the first 20 ms after a very brief click stimulus. One thousand or more sweeps are usually taken to average over time intervals as short as this, both because the changes in potential difference are so tiny and because no habituation or practice effects are assumed to occur. Jewett and Williston (1971) identified five reliably occurring positive peaks in the first 10 ms of the AEP, suggesting that they could be generated in the acoustic nerve, the cochlear nucleus, the superior olive, the lateral lemniscus and the inferior colliculus, respectively (see Figure 3.2). The peaks labelled VI and VII in Figure 3.2 were present for some subjects, not for others. Goff *et al.* (1977), using implanted electrode recordings, confirmed that some of the activity in the first 10 ms after an auditory signal originates in the lemniscal nucleus, but found that the slightly later components between 10 and 20 ms were irretrievably contaminated by muscle activity — which obscured the activity which would otherwise be expected from the primary cortex. As they said, it seems paradoxical that it is possible to record brainstem activity from the scalp, but no primary cortex activity. Electrical potentials generated by the muscle activity associated with hearing were so pervasive that even depth probes in Heschl's gyrus in the temporal lobe could not resolve primary cortical responses.

Somatosensory evoked potentials (SEPs) are normally elicited by applying an electric shock either to the skin or directly to a nerve. Allison *et al.* (1983) used the median nerve at the level of the wrist, finding that a clear positive peak could be detected at the shoulder, reflecting the nerve's compound action potential, with an 11 ms latency, arriving between 3 and 5 ms later as presynaptic afferent volleys at the spinal cord. Recordings from contralateral parietal scalp locations (P3 and P4) showed a sizeable (2 μV) waveform with a large negative peak at about 20 ms, which has been identified as reflecting somatosensory cortex activity.

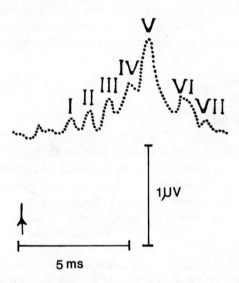

Figure 3.2 Auditory far field (brainstem) potential, averaged from 1000 sweeps, 2 click stimuli per second. From Jewett and Williston (1971)

These very early EP components could be used to index peripheral auditory and somatosensory processing, and have potential applications in the investigation of sensory coding. They have already been used in clinical assessment in neurology. Markand *et al.* (1980), for instance, found the brainstem auditory potential a useful test, complementing the EEG in the diagnosis of chronic central nervous system degenerative diseases in that it gives a specific assessment of brainstem function, allowing of the differentiation between various degenerative disorders. In addition, brainstem potentials have been used to evaluate coma and brain death. Starr (1977), in a study of 22 patients with isoelectric EEGs, found that while wave I could persist or even become exaggerated, the other brainstem potentials' components were absent. As he pointed out, this cannot be used as a definitive test of brain death, since deafness would render it useless. However, in conjunction with other information (for instance, from longer-latency visual evoked responses) it could be usefully informative.

Subcortical Gating

An issue of enduring interest to psychologists and neurophysiologists is whether any attentional processing can go on at a subcortical level. Hernandez-Peon (1966) suggested that listening could be suppressed at a peripheral level in the cat in favour of looking. That is, the nerve impulses caused by sound do not even reach the cortex but are suppressed peripherally as the hungry animal's visual attention is engaged by the sight of a mouse. Despite suggestions that his recordings may have been contaminated by muscle activity in the ear, and that any inhibition of sensory input may be general rather than specific to one modality, subsequent work seems to confirm that subcortical gating can indeed occur (see, e.g., Oatman and Anderson, 1977).

Evoked potential evidence for this is still equivocal, however. Lukas (1980, 1981) reported reductions in very early components of the auditory evoked potential when subjects' visual attention was engaged, consistent with the notion that auditory information was being filtered at the receptor level. That is, the auditory nerve component of the brainstem potential, peaking about 2.25 ms after stimulus onset, was reduced. Although statistically significant, this effect was not an invariable correlate of attentional distraction — some subjects did not show the effect at all. Picton *et al.* (1981) failed to replicate these promising findings, and Lukas (1982) has suggested that shifts in arousal in some of his subjects may account for the lack of unanimity in the results. Experiments involving electric shock stimuli have shown no evidence for subcortical gating (Desmedt and Robertson, 1977; Velasco *et al.*, 1980). Perhaps their stimuli were just too imperatively painful to be blocked out with this mechanism! The evoked potential evidence is obviously not very strong on this issue. If peripheral auditory and somatosensory inhibition were a normal consequence of the engagement of visual attention, it would be very surprising if there were not an easily measurable evoked potential correlate. We have to conclude that although it is possible that the physiological mechanisms may exist for subcortical gating, their effective operation is fairly rare.

Visual Feature Analysis

Visual evoked potentials (VEPs) do not show this differentiation of very early components — the first clearly identifiable peak is the P100, reflecting visual cortical activity. However, VEPs to patterned stimuli are reliably different from those to unpatterned flash stimuli. Harter (1971) showed that there is a reversal of the polarity of the VEP between 100 and 120 ms to patterned stimuli. He avoided confounding the effect of patterning with changes in stimulus intensity by comparing focused with unfocused stimuli, so that the total amount of light delivered to the eye was the same, whether patterning was present or absent. This work is discussed more fully in the next section, on attentional processing, which includes an account of subsequent experiments which, he argued, showed that this component specifically reflects feature detection rather than object localisation in the visual system. (There is neurophysiological evidence that these two functions are served by different neural pathways.)

ATTENTIONAL PROCESSES

Spong *et al.* (1965) showed that event-related potentials were larger when they were responses to stimuli on a channel (vision or audition) to which the subject had been instructed to attend (see Figure 3.3). If, as this work suggests, it could be shown that perceptual processing was indexed by ERPs, this would provide a potentially important source of information about attentional processes.

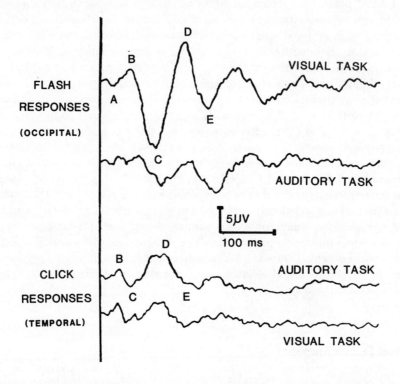

Figure 3.3 The effect of attention on the evoked potential. Occipital responses to flash stimuli (top two waveforms) are much greater when the subject is instructed to attend to visual stimuli. Similarly, temporal responses to click stimuli (bottom two waveforms) are greater when the subject is instructed to attend to auditory stimuli. From Spong *et al.* (1965)

Psychological models of attention have suggested that the cortical evaluation of stimuli may proceed in stages, so that a relatively low-level filter will select stimuli on the basis of physical characteristics (modality, frequency, amplitude, direction) and that subsequent further analysis depends to a greater or lesser extent on the outcome of early selection (Treisman, 1969; Broadbent, 1971). However, it is still unclear whether the low-level filters 'really' exist, or, if they do, whether they exclude or merely attenuate stimuli. If EEG reflects the operation of these processes, it would seem feasible to use EEG evidence to resolve some issues which are central to cognitive psychology.

Hillyard *et al.* (1973) attempted to identify not only the EEG *result* of an attentional process, but also the moment at which it occurred, and to link directly EEG evidence with the psychological filtering and selection processes hypothesised by Broadbent and Treisman. In their experiment, subjects were required to identify deviant stimuli, represented by a barely distinguishable shift in frequency, attending to one ear at a time (although stimuli were also presented to the non-attended ear for purposes of comparison). The fast rate of presentation used and the high level of difficulty of the task ensured that subjects were forced to attend carefully to the ear specified in the instructions, and the unpredictable timing of stimuli made anticipation difficult. The evidence of Hillyard *et al.* (see Figure 3.4) showed not only that the effects of attention were noticeable within one modality, but also that the event potential correlate of this early selection process was measurable as soon as 60 ms after the stimulus. They interpreted this evidence as showing that these changes in the N1 wave reflected the stimulus set of the subject, while a later positivity (at P300) was associated with stimulus detection.

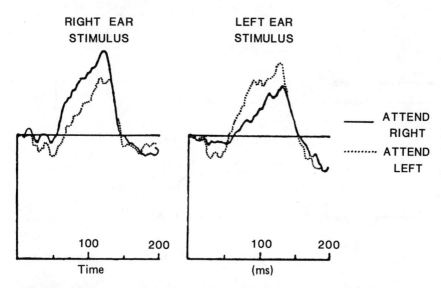

Figure 3.4 The effect of attention on the evoked potential. Vertex EPs are greater to attended stimuli than to unattended in the same modality (hearing) but presented to the unattended ear. From Hillyard *et al.* (1973)

Careful subsequent experimentation (Naatanen and Michie, 1979; Hansen and Hillyard, 1980) has shown that the N1 enhancement is due to a general negative shift, which can arise as early as 60 ms latency and which may persist for as long as 500 ms (see Figure 3.5). Its timing and amplitude are determined by parameters such as the signal interstimulus interval (ISI) and the difficulty of the detection task. Under some circumstances this 'processing negativity', as it has come to be called, does not appear until after the N1 component (see, e.g., Naatanen *et al.*, 1979). It is therefore unrealistic to link this component to stimulus selection alone. Naatanen (1982), in a definitive review of the huge amount of experimental evidence that has accumulated over a very short period of time, summarised the position in the following way: 'As far as the auditory and somatosensory modalities are concerned, when stimulus-category separation

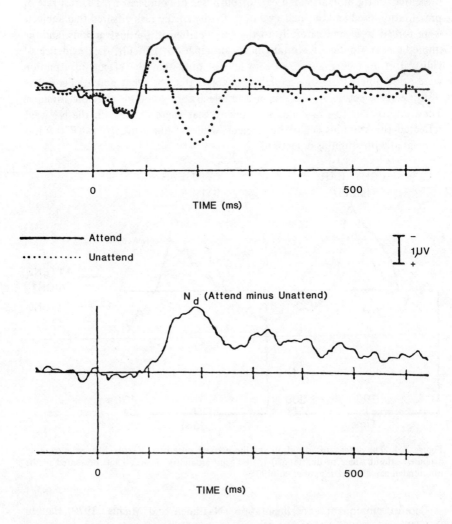

Figure 3.5 The effect of attention on the evoked potential. The difference between the EP to attended and unattended stimuli (N_d, the bottom waveform) is not confined to the first negative peak (N1) but is maintained for over 500 ms. From Hansen and Hillyard (1980)

is wide and variable ISIs are short, the processing negativity starts very early, overlapping the exogenous N1 component and enhancing its measured amplitudes. The processing negativity can even be observed with very small separations (e.g. 300 Hz vs 350 Hz in Hansen and Hillyard, 1980) when variable ISIs are short, but then its onset is delayed (and its topography is more posterior).'

He goes on to argue that processing negativity (Nd) has two components, the first of which reflects the identification of a stimulus as being a target for attention, and the second reflecting either further processing of the stimulus or a rehearsal of its characteristics. While it is clear that processing negativity indexes attentional and perceptual processes, it is not possible to identify particular, easily identifiable components with particular psychological processes. This line of research represents an example of the convergence of psychological and electroencephalographic research on some of the most intractable problems facing psychology. It is still being actively pursued.

A different line of attack on attentional processes is to use multidimensional criteria for stimulus selection. When searching for a particular stimulus (for instance, a red maple leaf) do we first identify any red object, and then evaluate its shape, or do we do the whole task all at once, using a template including all the relevant features?

It seems that in audition this depends largely on strategies used by subjects, determined by the relative difficulty of the discriminations. Hansen and Hillyard (1983) used auditory stimuli which varied in location (the variation being achieved with stereophonic headphones) and in frequency. Varying the difficulty of the discriminations along these two dimensions allowed them to assess an independent model of recognition (i.e. that, regardless of difficulty, the analysis of the two components of the task proceed independently) against a hierarchical model (in which the easier discrimination is dealt with first). Their results suggested that the easier discrimination is made first, and is only followed by the more difficult one if the first analysis was positive.

Using visual stimuli, Harter *et al.* (1979) required subjects to attend to gratings (rows of parallel lines) which differed in orientation and spacing. Early negative components appeared to follow identification of the two dimensions in sequence, and there was no indication that subjects' strategies had any effect on these components. Early visual selection is 'feature-specific'. Physiological evidence points to the visual system being organised into two distinct channels. One originates in the peripheral retina, is fast, projects onto the central cortex, and is involved in the location and orientation of stimuli. The other originates in the central retina of the eye, is slow, projects onto the occipital cortex and is a feature detection system. It would be unsurprising to find evoked potential correlates of the two systems. Hillyard and Munte (1984), in an experiment on the detection of red or blue stimuli, either 5 degrees left or right of a fixation spot, confirmed that initial selection always seemed to be based on location, and colour was subsequently ignored (from the EEG evidence) if the stimulus was in the 'wrong' place.

Further evoked potential evidence bearing on the issue of whether the two visual systems can operate and develop independently comes from some experiments reported by Neville *et al.* (1983). Normally we use our ears to attend to peripheral stimuli, and use the auditory system to direct our visual attention. However, people who have been deaf all their lives have to use peripheral visual cues for the same purpose. Will their visual systems have developed differently to compensate for the normal inadequacy of peripheral vision? Neville *et al.* found that, behaviourally, deaf subjects were extremely sensitive to peripheral visual stimuli (18 degrees from the centre), detecting them more reliably and quickly than hearing subjects, although their performance on centrally presented stimuli was about the same as that of hearing subjects. The deaf subjects' N150 was similar to that of hearing subjects for centrally presented stimuli, but the N150 enhancement by attention was much greater occipitally for deaf subjects. These findings suggest that some compensatory hypertrophy may have occurred in the visual system of deaf people as children to take over the functions normally undertaken by the auditory system.

These approaches to the problems of visual and auditory detection represent serious attempts to resolve issues in cognitive psychology by use of electrophysiological techniques and if the answers they offer are not definitive, they at least have shown the power of these techniques in addressing what are essentially problems in psychology. What is very clear from this work is that visual attentional processes are uniquely determined by the neurological substrate, and that no single grand psychological theory of attention will be able to deal with both audition and vision.

The Orienting Response

Every one is familiar with the experience of hearing a clock stopping ticking — an uncanny sensation, since one has normally not been listening to it, and, if asked, would probably have to pay attention to confirm whether the ticking was going on or not. Snyder and Hillyard (1976) investigated the N2 component in relation to unexpected stimuli, or changes in stimulation, confirming previous reports that it was greater to a deviant stimulus in a long series of identical auditory stimuli. Very significantly, they found that this N2 enhancement did not occur to infrequent stimuli. N2 enhancement does not occur if the deviant stimuli are presented more than 10 per cent of the time. The rate of stimulus presentation is also important, in that the enhancement will not appear if the interstimulus interval is greater than about 10 s, as if the 'usual' stimulus produced only a short-lived template. It was therefore argued that this component indexes the working of a mismatch detector, of the sort suggested by Sokolov 20 years earlier, in his theoretical treatment of the 'orienting response' (Sokolov, 1964).

There is evidence that is consistent with the identification of two components in N2 enhancement — which have been labelled 'mismatch negativity' and the

N2b. Naatanen and Gaillard (1983) summarised the relevant findings, which seem to show that the earlier component is a reflection of physical deviance *per se*, and is unaffected by any evaluation of the stimulus in terms of its significance or meaning. For instance, Naatanen *et al.* (1978) found that mismatch negativity occurred in response to infrequent oddball stimuli whether they were attended to or not. (Trains of stimuli were presented to both ears, and subjects were instructed to count the deviant stimuli in one or the other.) In another experiment, subjects instructed to read and ignore the stimuli showed mismatch negativity to deviant stimuli, although this was not followed by the positive component (P300) typical of responses to detected stimuli when subjects were counting them. They also report some previously unpublished data showing that deviant stimuli missed by a subject were followed by mismatch negativity which was not maintained for as long as that following detected stimuli, although it was of the same order of magnitude.

Whether it is divisible into two components or not, the N2 deflection does seem to reflect an orienting response, since it is insensitive to attentional demands. However, there are two important ways in which it differs from the orienting response (OR): first, while the classical OR is elicited by any stimulus for which a neuronal model does not exist, the N2 enhancement only occurs to a mismatch with an existing model; and second, as Naatanen and Gaillard point out, the distribution of the N2 on the scalp is inconsistent with its being generated in the hippocampus, the site that Sokolov has identified in the rabbit for the generation of the OR.

THE P300

Sutton *et al.* (1965) first reported this late positive wave following a stimulus which was apparently a consequence of the resolution of uncertainty. Subjects were required to guess which of two possible stimuli were about to occur. The evoked potential had the greater late positivity (at about 300 ms) the more improbable the stimulus. P300 amplitude was determined by its subjective probability (influenced, for instance, by the number of times it had been repeated recently) rather than its objective frequency (see Figure 3.6).

The P300 is not confined to auditory evoked potentials. Friedman *et al.* (1975) demonstrated that it could be elicited with printed words as stimuli, just as much as speech, when recording the evoked potential to the final word in an otherwise ambiguous sentence. The P300 component was only noticeable to the word which resolved the sentence ambiguity.

The P300 has been implicated in an almost embarrassingly large number of psychological processes, and seems remarkably unspecific. Its latency is frequently quoted as being 400 ms or more, and appears to be related to task difficulty. In fact, it is now conventional to represent P300 as P$\overline{300}$, to indicate the elasticity of its latency. The variability in P300 latency is the source of another problem in assessing amplitude, as the outcome of averaging a number of large positive waves is a rather shallow positive wave, which gives no true indication of the average amplitude of the EEG responses. This phenomenon, referred to as 'jitter' by encephalographers, can to some extent be overcome by the use of principal components analysis (PCA) as well as summation, but most of the published work on P300 has not included PCA or any other estimation of jitter.

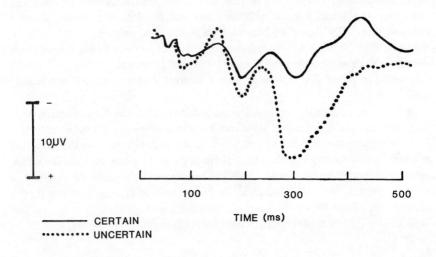

Figure 3.6 The P300. The solid tracing is the EP to sound stimuli which the subject was certain would be sounds; the dashed tracing is the EP to identical stimuli of whose sensory modality the subject was uncertain. Stimuli resolving uncertainty typically elicit a positive-going component which reaches peak amplitude at about 300 ms. From Sutton *et al.* (1965)

Sutton (1982), in a lecture reviewing the evidence accumulated over 18 years, rather wryly said that it gave him six impossible things to believe before breakfast. Informational value, task relevance and whether the stimulus is a target or not all affect P300. Paradoxically, the P300 can be larger for uninformative feedback, or larger for entirely predictable stimuli (when fairly rare). Could there be at least two different components involved here, with fairly similar latencies? Sutton suggested that the P300 elicited by expected, task-relevant stimuli is more parietal in origin, while that produced by surprising or novel stimuli is frontal, and another manifestation of the orienting response.

This component of the evoked potential therefore conforms to Regan's (1972) criteria for an endogenous component more than any other, in being entirely a reflection of the evaluation of a signal rather than a response to it. Evaluation implies attention to the signal but also something else — the assessment of meaning, in terms of what the signal may denote, its connotations and associations. Some psychologists have been arguing for the past 10 years that the single most important determinant of the memorability of an item in a list is the 'depth' of processing to which it is subjected — the degree to which its meaning has been explored (see, e.g., Craik and Lockhardt, 1972). Donchin (1981) has followed this up by assuming that P300 amplitude reflects the evaluative processing necessary for ensuring an enduring memory trace. If this were true, it should be possible to predict which items in a list of words are most memorable from the amplitude of the P300 responses elicited from them when first presented. That is, the bigger the P300 amplitude when an item was presented, the greater the 'depth' of processing. The success of this and subsequent experiments (Karis *et al.*, 1984) has been part of the challenge issued to other encephalographers referred to at the beginning of this chapter, and it certainly takes the rather refined laboratory techniques of encephalography back into the realm of experimental psychology.

The Origin of the P300

Halgren *et al.* (1980) took advantage of the opportunity to study six epileptic patients who had implanted electrodes in their mid-brains. Recording simultaneously from the scalp and intracranially, they found similar waveforms deep in the hippocampus of greater amplitude with the same latency as those on the scalp, which led them to suggest that the P300 is generated in the hippocampus itself. The hippocampus is anatomically placed in the centre of the limbic system, and damage to it commonly results in memory impairment in human beings (see, e.g., Weiskrantz and Warrington, 1975). Animal experimentation suggests that it has an important part to play in the regulation of attentional processes. Its identification as the source of the P300 could therefore be interpreted as providing support for Donchin's theory of the functions that the waveform indexes — the updating of memory through attentional processing.

Subcortical recordings have also been made from a single patient suffering from intractable pain from a back injury, who had electrodes implanted in the right somatosensory thalamus and bilaterally in the hindbrain, by Yingling and Hosobuchi (1984). They found that the rare auditory and visual stimuli accompanied by a P300 at the scalp were also accompanied by negative activity at the subcortical sites, and argued that this is inconsistent with a hippocampal generator for the P300, suggesting instead that it reflects the attentional processing which has previously been attributed to the thalamus. Clinical findings such as these must always be regarded as somewhat tentative, relying on fortuitous observations in patients who are inevitably in poor health. All the same, the apparent ubiquity of 300 ms activity following a rare stimulus reinforces the impression that it does not index any single process. Donchin's theory must be regarded as not proven.

P300 and Workload

Before dealing with the evidence linking the P300 with workload, or attentional resource allocation, it may be appropriate to summarise the behavioural evidence on workload estimation, for the reader unfamiliar with this branch of ergonomics. There have been a number of attempts to measure how hard an individual may be working, both from the point of view of making sure that workers are not idling and, more interestingly, to assess the amount of effective workload that an operator can handle without performance breaking down. This becomes particularly important in the context of extensive control systems – for instance, in the chemical and petrochemical industry, where potentially dangerous processes are remotely controlled, and, of course, in the highly demanding roles of aircraft pilot or air traffic controller.

One of the most effective ways of estimating workload is to provide the operator with a secondary task, in addition to his or her 'normal' work, and to measure how much of the secondary task gets completed under different conditions. Secondary task performance is then presumed to be a measure of 'spare' mental capacity. Brown (1961) used it to investigate the effect of radio-telephones on driving, asking subjects to answer questions on the telephone while driving through gaps of varying sizes. Accuracy and latency in answering questions was affected by having to drive at the same time, but not in proportion to difficulty level of the primary (driving) task. However, telephoning did impair judgements of 'impossible' tasks – drivers attempted to negotiate gaps which were narrower than the car when they had to answer the telephone at the same time. This technique obviously has its limitations, and one would hesitate before asking an aircraft pilot, for instance, to answer lots of irrelevant questions while landing an aircraft in order to assess any residual mental capacity!

An ideal method of measuring workload should be unobtrusive and yet sensitive. Simple physiological measures of heart rate, skin conductance, pupil dilation and respiration tend to reflect changes in arousal, which may be determined as much by the importance of a task as by its difficulty. The P300 has all the advantages of being an involuntary response, and is also determined by the degree of cognitive processing or evaluation of the signal that it follows. Wickens *et al.* (1977) and Isreal *et al.* (1980) have attempted to harness these interesting properties to workload measurement. Their primary task was two-dimensional tracking, in which subjects manipulated a control stick with their right hand and attempted to hold an error cursor within a reference target in the middle of a CRT display. This tracking could be made more or less difficult. The secondary task was to count the number of tones at a certain pitch, ignoring an equal number of other tones. They found that the amplitude of the P300 to the attended tones was reduced by having a concurrent task (the tracking task), although increasing the task difficulty did not further reduce P300 amplitude.

Wickens *et al.* (1983) have refined the technique further, embedding flash stimuli in the primary tracking task display as the secondary task probes, so as to index the same perceptual resource with both tasks. With this procedure they succeeded in demonstrating a decrease in P300 amplitude with increasing difficulty of tracking, showing that it is indeed feasible to assess workload relatively unobtrusively, as long as an appropriate secondary task can be found. Wickens *et al.* return to Donchin's (1981) model of P300 as being involved primarily in the updating of working memory in explaining their results, and argue that the limit in resources lies in the 'updating subroutine' rather than in the act of perception itself or in attentional switching.

Just how practicable is this technique in workload assessment? Two industrial psychology postgraduates in Hull (Giannocourou, 1984; Kluvitse, 1984) attempted to replicate one of the early experiments, using a visual tracking task of variable difficulty and a secondary auditory counting task. Their aim was mainly to estimate the ease with which workload could be assessed in an applied setting. While their results confirmed the general finding that P300 was decreased by the addition of a secondary task, it was clear that the reliability of the effect depended on extremely careful matching of the two tasks in terms of level of difficulty. It is unlikely that this method of workload assessment will be useful in any but the most exotic technological settings, such as the development of aircraft control systems.

SLOW POTENTIALS

Bereitschaftspotentials (BPs) and the contingent negative variation (CNV) were discovered at about the same time, by Kornhuber and Deecke (1965) and Walter *et al.* (1964), respectively. Oddly enough, very little effort was made for the first 10 years after their discovery to come to an integrated understanding of these two very similar waveforms, which both precede movement. In this section an attempt will be made to do this.

Bereitschaftspotentials

The BP is a negative potential over central areas of the scalp which precedes voluntary movement. Typically, a subject is instructed to press a button 'every few seconds'. No stimuli are presented, and averaging is done with respect to the response. McAdam and Seales (1969) confirmed that this waveform, beginning about 1000 ms before movement, was asymmetrically distributed with greater negativity contralaterally (as one might expect, if the BP does indeed index motor cortex function). They also manipulated motivational levels in their subjects by randomly sounding a buzzer in one condition on half the trials which indicated that the subject was 'correct' and would receive 10 cents. In the control condition the buzzer always sounded when the subject pressed the button, but it did not indicate a 10 cent reward. The BP amplitude was approximately doubled in the rewarded condition, from 8 to 16 μV on the contralateral side and from 4 to 8 μV ipsilaterally (see Figure 3.7).

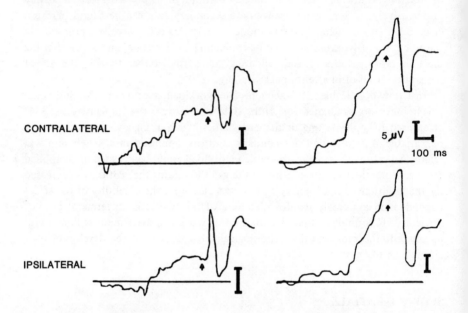

Figure 3.7 Bereitschaftspotentials (BPs). Negativity develops on the scalp before a response (indicated by the arrows). It is greater contralaterally than ipsilaterally (upper versus lower traces) and is greater when the response may be rewarded than when there is no such possibility (right versus left traces). From McAdam and Seales (1969)

The effects of reward are really rather incalculable. A similar experiment by Kutas and Donchin (1977) simply required subjects to vary the force exerted in making the response. The BP was the greater the more forceful the response anticipated. One could interpret both these results in terms of the amount of effort the subject was putting into the response, either mental (in guessing whether the response was going to be rewarded or not) or physical. McAdam and Seales did not measure the amount of force exerted by their subjects, which is a pity; quite possibly, the rewarded subjects made more forceful responses.

Many motor responses are not anticipated by as much as a second – the simple reaction time, for instance, is normally faster than 200 ms, so the BP is obviously not essential to movement, in its fully developed form. Libet *et al.* (1983a) instructed a subject to plan to make a movement when a revolving light arrived at a certain point, but then to 'veto' this intention at a point in the light's orbit which was about 150 ms before it would have reached the original 'movement point'. Even this spurious intention to act resulted in a slow negative wave developing on the scalp, indistinguishable from a 'real' BP. If, however, the subject was instructed merely to anticipate the moment when the light reached a certain point, this did not result in any negative shift. Libet *et al.* interpreted this evidence as supporting the notion that both BPs and CNVs only accompany intentions to act, whether an action is ultimately called for or not. In another experiment using the same experimental set-up, Libet *et al.* (1983b) asked subjects to report when they first began intending to act, finding that the onset of measurable cerebral activity clearly preceded it by several hundred milli-seconds. The cerebral initiation of a spontaneous, freely voluntary act can there-fore begin unconsciously.

Contingent Negative Variation

The CNV, or expectancy wave, is defined in terms of an experimental paradigm. A warning stimulus (S1) is followed after an interstimulus interval (ISI) of between 1 and 3 s by an imperative stimulus (S2) to which the subject is normally required to make a response. During the ISI a ramp-like negative potential is generated on the scalp which is resolved after the IS and consequent response. (See Figure 3.8.)

The whole waveform must be a composite of at least two components – the ERP to S1 and the ramp-like negative wave. Is this all, and is the CNV really totally different from the BP, despite both of them having a similar appearance and both normally preceding a simple movement? Like the BP, the CNV increases with motivational level. However, it is normally assumed to be symmetrically distributed, and, more important, it is not essential for a response to be made to S2 for a CNV waveform to be generated, merely that the stimulus should be anticipated (ensured, for instance, by accompanying it with an electric shock). It is thus clear that the BP and CNV are not identical, but the possibility remains that one or both of them are composite waveforms and that they share one or more component. CNV experiments in which the ISI is lengthened to 3 s (see, e.g., Loveless and Sanford, 1974) show that there is an early negativity which develops frontally on the scalp in the first second of the ISI, followed by a second ramp-like component beginning about 1 s before S2, centred on the vertex. Loveless and Sanford suggested that the CNV could be analysed into two com-ponents – an orienting response following the warning stimulus (S1) and an expectancy wave preceding S2. (It should be noted here that this usage of 'orienting response' is by no means as precise as that used in the context of mismatch negativity and N2 enhancement. Gaillard (1980) has suggested calling this early CNV component a slow negative wave (SNW). This would distinguish it from N2 and remove the possibly misleading connotation to the OR.)

Even if we accept that the CNV is made up of these two components (and opinion is not unanimous on the subject) the question still remains: is the so-called expectancy component really different from the BP? Gaillard (1977) addressed this issue by distinguishing expectancy from mere motor preparation.

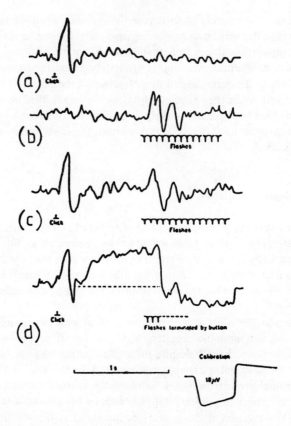

Figure 3.8 The contingent negative variation (CNV). Averages of responses to 12 presentations. (a) Response in frontovertical region to clicks; (b) flicker; (c) clicks followed by flicker; (d) clicks followed by flicker terminated by the subject pressing a button as instructed. From Walter *et al.* (1964)

In his experiment S1 informed the subject of the probability of S2 being presented at all — 0.9, 0.5 or 0 — thus providing three levels of expectancy. Motor preparation was varied by instructing subjects either to respond as *fast* as possible, to respond as *accurately* as possible or to delay their response by 1 s after the IS. The ISI again was 3 s — unusually long for a CNV experiment, but essential if the two components are to be distinguished. Gaillard found that the late negativity immediately preceding S2 disappeared if an immediate response was not required, suggesting that this component may indeed share a good deal with the BP. The early negativity was more frontal than central and parietal, and was relatively insensitive to whether a response was required immediately, or whether instructions for speed or accuracy had been given. This evidence is consistent with the suggestion that the early CNV is a cortical component of an orienting response, and also that the later component, the expectancy wave, may be identical with the component called the BP.

Following up this work, Gaillard and Perdok (1980) manipulated the inform-ative value of S1 by varying its pitch — it either warned the subject that he or she should respond as quickly as possible, even at the cost of some errors, or as *accurately* as possible, without making any error, or, thirdly, simply announced the imminent arrival of S2, without any implicit instruction. When S1 was informative, the amplitude of CNV in the first 2 s was elevated, while there was no difference between conditions in amplitude of the ramp-like negativity immediately preceding S2. Gaillard (1980) argued that the first component, which he called the slow negative wave (SNW), is dependent on the characteristics of S1 in the same way as the P300 is determined by the informational value of the stimulus. In contrast, the terminal CNV is determined merely by level of motor preparation.

SUMMING UP

A number of attempts are being and have been made to use identifiable com-ponents in dealing with psychological issues. The modest successes achieved so far have made it clear that the whole enterprise is not doomed, and that Donchin's challenge, referred to at the beginning of the chapter, may one day be met.

Exogenous components have a readily recognisable signature, definable in peak latency, in their distribution over the scalp and their amplitude. A simplistic approach would be to attempt to treat endogenous components in the same way — identifying components by their signature and then investigating them in terms of psychological determinants, making the assumption that a particular psychological process is always mirrored in a particular waveform. However, endogenous components are not so obligingly transparent, varying in response time and amplitude for sometimes unpredictable reasons. Gaillard and Verduin (1985) suggest that since there is no simple way of recognising endogenous components by latency, amplitude or shape, the criteria for defining them should be a combination of their scalp distribution, reflecting their underlying neurophysiology, and the psychological factors determining their occurrence. Naturally, this is a somewhat ambiguous model of event-related components (compared with the one implicit from exogenous component analysis), but perhaps more realistic.

4

EEG and Localisation of Function in the Brain

RUNNING EEG

Ever since Caton's experiments in the 1870s, it has been one of the preoccupations of encephalographers to identify localised brain functions. Adrian and Yamigawa's rather macabre experiment (described in Chapter 1) on the dipole placed in a corpse showed that fairly precise triangulation of localised electrical activity deep in the brain is possible from electrodes on the scalp. The clinical application of EEG, of course, quite routinely depends on this in the localisation of foreign bodies, tumours and epileptic foci. In the modern experimental context, the object of identifying correlates of localised functions must be to make EEG evidence available in the analysis of normal functioning. As with event-related potentials, the mere correlation of EEG phenomena with known brain functions is uninteresting in itself, but is an essential first step towards realising this ambition.

Running Alpha Asymmetry

The origin of the alpha rhythm, distributed over the occipital cortex, has already been discussed at some length in Chapter 1. It clearly emanates from the cortex, rather than peripherally. While it is still uncertain whether it directly indexes visual function, it would be uncontentious to state that its appearance and blocking is largely controlled by the visual system. The auditory modality does not have any specific analogous EEG correlate, which reflects the low neurological investment in audition in man, compared with the one-third of all afferent tissue which is visual in origin.

The obvious way of assessing localisation of brain function through EEG is to compare the amplitude of the dominant rhythm – the alpha rhythm – recorded from the two sides of the head. Clinical evidence strongly suggests that the hemispheres are not identical in function. Damage to the left hemisphere typically results in disorders related to language, and during the nineteenth century neurologists identified two areas — called Broca's area and Wernicke's area, after the clinicians who first drew attention to them — which appear to be crucial to the production and understanding of speech (see Figure 4.1). This evidence of specialisation and the apparent lack of a specific function for the right hemisphere naturally suggested that the left was more important. Hughlings Jackson (Taylor, 1958) first articulated the idea of cerebral 'dominance', that the left hemisphere is somehow in charge in right-handed individuals, while the right, or 'minor', hemisphere performs a subsidiary role.

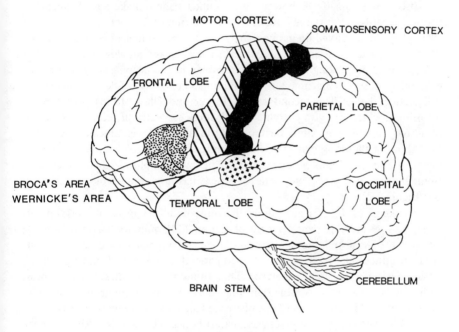

Figure 4.1 The left hemisphere

Taking this idea fairly literally, one might expect a more active, low-voltage EEG on the left-hand side in right-handers. This sounds like a simple and easily tested proposition, and there have been a number of studies of EEG asymmetry in normal people, but they do not provide a simple, easily stated answer. The following account is not a definitive review of all the experiments published on this topic, but concentrates on those which illustrate some of the difficulties faced by encephalographers, and the ones which have to some extent surmounted the difficulties.

Visual analysis of the EEG of relaxed right-handed subjects suggests no overall asymmetry in alpha abundance. However, there are local variations, and while there are no differences in alpha abundance between left and right occipital areas, greater abundance is noticeable at the right parietal regions than at the left, and the reverse in central and temporal regions (Bell and Van Ireland, 1976). These results — all statistically significant — were based on monopolar recordings.

Fourier (frequency) analysis of bipolar recordings gives a very different picture. Butler and Glass (1976) reported greater combined EEG amplitude (of all frequencies) over the right hemisphere than over the left in both left-handed and right-handed subjects. Alpha amplitude was the same over the two hemispheres in relaxed subjects, regardless of handedness.

The first of these studies suffers from the handicap of using visual analysis of the EEG — the human eye, however well trained, cannot make reliable quantitative judgements about the relative amounts of different frequencies of waveform when they are all mixed up in one signal, and is liable to make systematic errors. (Particular patterns of activity, however, such as spike and slow wave, which a clinician may be looking for, or the K complex in the sleeping subject, are very difficult to define in machine terms, and human beings have a decided advantage in spotting them.) The second study (Butler and Glass, 1976) used bipolar recordings, which can give extremely misleading estimates of relative amplitude of activity at different sites. Beaumont (1983) has very graphically illustrated this, showing that a bipolar recording from, for instance, two active sites whose signals are in phase can produce an EEG of lower amplitude than a recording from another two sites, only one of which has any appreciable signal at all (see Figure 4.2).

Wieneke *et al.* (1980) have done the most definitive piece of work on this issue, in size and representativeness of sample (110 military servicemen being assessed for flying training) and methodology (monopolar recordings from four sites on either side, referenced to fronto-parietal locations Fp1 and Fp2, using both spectral and coherence analysis). They found that, regardless of handedness, alpha tends to be greater on the right than the left in all locations, but especially between P3 and P4 and T5 and T6. Coherence (the correlation between frequency spectra) between the hemispheres was greatest between O1 and O2. All coherence measures within hemispheres were greater than those between hemispheres. This confirms that EEG is generated independently in the two hemispheres, and, given the dominance of alpha rhythm in the occipital regions, where their coherence was greatest, the presence of two independent alpha generators.

Rolandic Wicket Rhythm

The Rolandic wicket rhythm, or 'mu' rhythm, was first described by Gastaut (1952) as being in the alpha frequency band, but localised on central areas of the scalp. It is blocked by movement of the contralateral hand, but not by the eyes being open, which indicates that it may genuinely reflect activity in the motor cortex, approximately underlying these electrode locations.

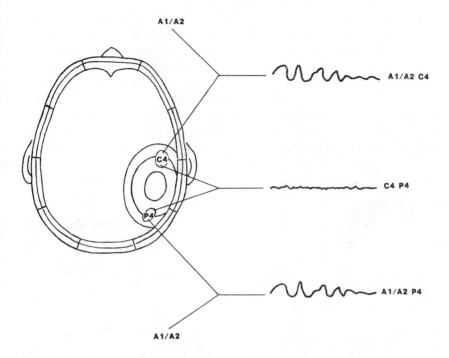

Figure 4.2 Electrode derivations. With electrodes astride a focus of activity (shown in concentric circles) the resulting bipolar recording (middle waveform) may show no evidence of it, while mastoid-referenced monopolar recordings (top and bottom waveforms) do so

Relatively few investigations of motor functioning have been done using this EEG component in human subjects, compared with the number of studies of the sensorimotor rhythms in animals such as the cat. This is − partly, at least − because it is somewhat elusive, with only a proportion of subjects displaying it at all, and also because it shares a frequency band with the rather pervasive alpha rhythm. Kuhlman (1980) confirmed Gastaut's observations on the mu rhythm, using spectral frequency analysis from occipital and central sites simultaneously, showing that alpha activity was not significantly reduced by movement so long as the eyes were shut, while mu activity, of lower amplitude than alpha, was significantly attenuated by movement. The rhythms could be distinguished, not only by location of maximal amplitude (occipital for alpha and central for mu), but also by a slightly faster peak frequency for mu than for alpha. Figure 4.3 shows frequency spectra from an individual subject selected for his relatively persistent alpha rhythm and unusually pronounced Rolandic rhythms, recorded in the Hull laboratory. Left and right central electrodes (C3 and C4) and the occipital derivation (O1) were referenced to linked mastoids. Occipital alpha was clearly attenuated by eye opening and by mental arithmetic performed with the eyes shut, while the centrally recorded EEG spectra continued to show pronounced mu activity at 10 Hz, which was itself attenuated by finger movements.

Does the blocking of mu reflect processes essential to the generation of voluntary movement? Probably not, as it has been reported that involuntary movements also attenuate the mu rhythm (Chatrian *et al.*, 1959) as well as somatosensory (electric shock) stimulation (Broughton *et al.*, 1964). (See Chatrian, 1976, for a definitive review.) Kuhlman suggests that the blocking of mu preceding movement is not directly related to motor processes. Rather, mu originates in the resting somatosensory cortex, and attenuation before movement

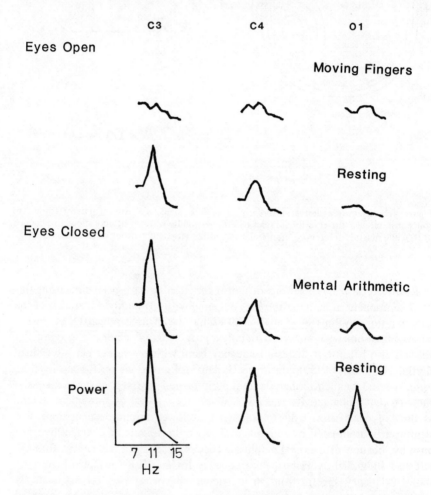

Figure 4.3 Rolandic and occipital frequency spectra. Persistent 10 Hz activity at C3 and C4 in this subject is only blocked by movement, while alpha activity recorded occipitally is blocked by mental arithmetic with eyes closed, and when the eyes are open

is evidence of the cortex becoming prepared to receive the afferent feedback which invariably results from movement. This neatly explains the evidence about involuntary movement and stimulation blocking mu. Reafference would normally be to the contralateral hemisphere, just as much as motor outflow is from the contralateral hemisphere, thus accounting for the asymmetry in mu blocking.

HEMISPHERICITY AND TASK-RELATED ASYMMETRY

As was stated in the last section, it has been known since the middle of the nineteenth century that damage to the left hemisphere in the adult commonly results in aphasia, or loss of speech, while damage to the right-hand side of the brain does not.

Very rarely, it is clinically necessary to separate the two halves of the brain in a patient by cutting the corpus callosum and other connections between the hemispheres, usually in order to control major epileptic seizures. Interest in hemisphere differences became intense during the 1970s, when it became clear that in these commissurotomised patients with 'split brains' the hemisphere could operate in complete independence without obvious behavioural consequences. Only rather subtle testing using the presentation of stimuli independently to the far left or right of the visual field (projecting to the visual cortex on the same side) elicited clear evidence for a dissociation of consciousness between the two sides of the brain. The patients could describe stimuli which were allowed to reach the left hemisphere, but could not describe the stimuli when they were presented so that they could only reach the right hemisphere. They could, however, draw stimuli which had only reached the right hemisphere. The left brain was thus found to be more articulate, and the right brain (the 'minor' hemisphere) relatively inarticulate but skilled in pattern perception and spatial analysis.

Since patients with bisected brains showed so few readily apparent signs of 'split consciousness' or any other obvious aberrations, could it be that the hemispheres normally operate in tandem and in relative independence? Could the two halves of the brain be responsible for different aspects of skill, and even of personality and style of thinking? It had always been assumed that the intact brain operated in a unified way, with the minor hemisphere adopting a relatively unimportant role. It now appeared that there might be an unsuspected degree of structural specialisation.

Just as in the studies on split-brain patients, experiments on normal subjects' response times to stimuli presented to left and right visual fields showed a clear left visual field advantage for words and a right visual field advantage for unfamiliar faces (Beaumont, 1981). Figure 4.4 may clarify this relationship between visual and cortical fields. These behavioural findings confirmed the clinical and neurophysiological evidence that the left hemisphere in right-handed people is more crucially involved in linguistic functioning than the right, also validating

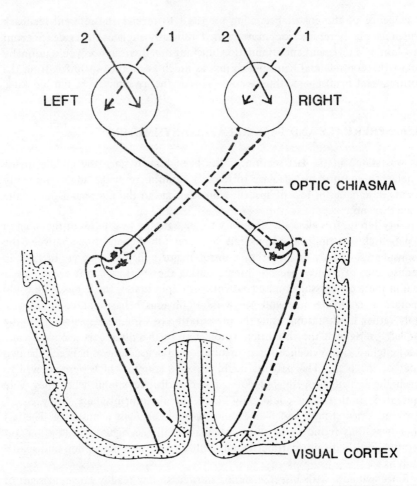

Figure 4.4 The visual system. Connections in the optic chiasma direct input from the right visual field in both eyes to the left visual cortex, and vice versa

the notion that hemispheric specialisation is usual in the intact brain. Most important for the last point was the actual advantage enjoyed by the right hemisphere in dealing with unfamiliar faces, suggesting that the idea of 'dominance' is inadequate to describe the functional specialisation of the two hemispheres in normal people with intact brains. The rather subtle differences between hemispheres' abilities has been summarised by Levy (1974) in a general description based on information processing style — briefly, that the left hemisphere's style is analytic, compared with a more holistic response pattern adopted by the right hemisphere. A description of one hemisphere being dominant and the other merely subservient is evidently inadequate to do justice to the differences in function which this research suggests.

A very large number of studies relating EEG asymmetry to the type of task in which the subject is involved have also generally indicated that the performance of verbal tasks is associated with left hemisphere activation, and that the performance of non-verbal, spatial or musical tasks is associated with right hemisphere activation. Again, a definitive review is not attempted here, but illustrative experiments will be described which show how much can be and has been achieved. The first report of task-related differences in EEG between the hemispheres was published in 1957 by Wilson *et al*. They found that writing on an imaginary blackboard produced more occipital alpha blocking in the left hemisphere than in the right, while the blocking produced by sounding a loud gong every 10 s was the same on both sides.

Subsequent experiments have varied in the extent to which they have improved on this one. McKee *et al*. (1973) showed that the ratio of alpha amplitude between left and right hemispheres depended on task, was sensitive to task difficulty and was independent of the total amount of alpha. In the verbal task, targets of increasing semantic complexity buried in a text were read out loud, so that the same material could be used for all conditions, and only the instructions to subjects had to be varied. The non-verbal task was a musical one, in which subjects were instructed to press a hand-held button whenever a particular theme in a Bach concerto was repeated. Increasing the difficulty of a verbal task decreased the total amount of alpha being produced.

Not all experiments have produced such clear-cut results, although it has generally been confirmed that the ratio of alpha activity between hemispheres is responsive to type of task. A critical review by Donchin *et al*. (1977) focused on the use of these ratio scores, which they said were potentially misleading. A change in ratio could be the result of a change in numerator, denominator, or both. Resting levels of asymmetry tend to be ignored, with researchers concentrating on ratios of asymmetry to the exclusion of other aspects of EEG, which could be equally relevant. A very important issue is whether these changes reflect actual structurally determined asymmetries in function or rather changes in subjects' strategies in dealing with task requirements. Graded levels of asymmetry in EEG activation according to gradations of task difficulty would be persuasive evidence for structural specialisation. Evidence is as yet inconclusive on this point.

Beaumont's observation about the importance of using monopolar recordings in the assessment of localisation of function is, of course, relevant to these studies as well as to those addressed to assessing resting levels of asymmetry. A good number of published studies have, in fact, used bipolar montages. In addition, it is misleading to assume that the careful use of left- and right-hand sites, indicated by the standard 10–20 system of electrode placement, will result in symmetrical placements with respect to the underlying cortical structures. There are, it seems, gross anatomical asymmetries in the surface of the brain, especially in temporal and parietal regions. As Beaumont has pointed out, it is perhaps not merely a coincidence that most of the studies which have reported asymmetries have recorded activity from such sites, inevitably confounding anatomical asymmetry with task effects.

On the other hand, it would be a mistake to dismiss all the evidence merely in the interests of methodological purity, and even Donchin *et al.* admit that 'there is a thread of positive results that indicate the promise of the approach'. Potentially a more damaging critique of these experiments was made by Gevins *et al.* (1979), arguing that the studies which were successful in demonstrating EEG correlates of hemisphericity all confounded motor task demands with cognitive demands. It now seems that this observation may not discredit the whole body of work, and indeed has added to our understanding, in that Yingling (1980) has shown that while it is true that only studies involving a motor component have produced positive results, this is independent of whether or not they controlled for any artefactual motor effects. That is, the EEG effects reported were 'real' to the extent that they were not by-products of the electrical signs of muscular activity, and task-dependent asymmetries do not occur merely with cogitation but only when action is involved. As Yingling says: '. . . the brain is organized to carry out its primary function of behaviour, not perception or cognition alone, and ... this primacy of action is reflected in the results of EEG studies of functional hemispheric asymmetry.'

Despite all this debate about methodological issues, and the publication of criteria for the acceptability of laboratory techniques, work continues to be published which shows little sign of having benefited from it. Loring and Sheer (1984), for instance, report a study on asymmetries in the distribution of 40 Hz activity during periods of concentrated attention on tasks of different sorts. Bipolar EEG montages were used, ratios of 40 Hz activity were given with no indication of the levels, and no attempt was made to match the verbal and spatial tasks for difficulty — three practices which have been repeatedly decried by Donchin *et al.* and Beaumont.

The 'hemisphericity' debate has also become the vehicle for a number of the more ill-defined if not woolly-minded modern notions — so that the right hemisphere has been equated with 'alternative' consciousness, lateral thinking, creativity and the unconscious mind itself. Sutherland (1985) has expressed this point with some wit: 'There is a popular belief that the right side of the brain is imaginative, intuitive, spontaneous, holistic, emotional and impulsive, while the left side is cold, calculating, analytic and objective. It has even been proposed that the problems of Western civilisation arise because its denizens use the left side of their brain too much and that the remedy lies in developing the other side, through devices such as encounter groups, pot, and liberated sex.'

Among the very large number of experiments reported on hemisphericity and running EEG, there have been a number which have been methodologically wanting — probably a greater proportion than in other areas, with the topicality of the subject-matter attracting some experimentalists with inadequate technical expertise. While EEG studies have, in general, confirmed the neurological and behavioural evidence referred to at the beginning of this section, they have usually not succeeded in taking the matter very much further. This is not only because of limitations on the EEG side, but also because of some lack of precision in defining the skills in which the two hemispheres are supposed to specialise and devising tasks of comparable levels of difficulty. The impatience of some of the erstwhile exponents of hemisphericity, such as Gevins or Beaumont, becomes understandable. However, two long-standing ideas about brain function have been discredited by the debate — the notion of cerebral dominance, with the minor hemisphere having little or no role in normal functioning, and the so-called 'law of mass action', which stated that the brain acts as a whole, with little or no localisation of function.

Hemisphericity and Evoked Potential Asymmetry

As with the running EEG experiments, attention has focused on the correlates of linguistic processing. In the first place, can the evoked potential distinguish linguistic stimulus materials from other stimuli? Second, can it differentiate different linguistic stimuli?

In a recent review Molfese (1983) criticises many of the very large number of studies done by a wide variety of individuals for being unsystematic, using linguistically unsophisticated stimuli and often only two electrode sites. The most telling criticism was his observation of the general preoccupation with demonstrating lateralised differences in evoked potentials, to the exclusion of any analysis of other evoked potential correlates of linguistic processing. Rugg (1983), reviewing the experimental work on high-level, meaningful material and lateralised evoked potentials, is similarly highly critical. He identifies the major reason for the failure to produce a coherent body of knowledge in this area as the lack of definition of task requirements which should produce asymmetrical processing. Other major problems are the wide variety of tasks used by different experimenters, and the large number of methodologically suspect studies. (Too many of the experiments represent isolated forays into the EEG undergrowth by individuals who then move on to other more tractable research problems.)

Rather than deal with this large and somewhat disappointing literature in detail, this section will concentrate on one line of enquiry which seems to be yielding some useful results. This is represented by Molfese's own work, which has confirmed that the auditory evoked potential does indeed distinguish speech from non-speech stimuli, in that the N1 component is asymmetrically distributed to speech stimuli, being greater on the left. A large number of other studies have also shown this effect, using a variety of non-linguistic and linguistic stimuli. Could there be something acoustically special or different about speech? Molfese set out to discover what was special about perception of the spoken word, concentrating on voice onset times of the bilabial stop consonants /b and p/ in the phonetics /ba/ and /pa/.

The voice onset time (VOT) is the delay between the beginning of an utterance with sound being generated in the larynx and the parting of the lips to release a burst of air. The main difference between the phonetics /pa/ and /ba/ is in the timing of the initial voicing, so that the VOT is briefer for /ba/ (less than 20 ms) than for /pa/. The discrimination of these rather fine distinctions is obviously vital to the comprehension of spoken language. Using principal components analysis based on individual EEG responses as well as analysis of variance of averaged components, Molfese demonstrated that components of the left hemisphere auditory evoked potential differentiate 0 from 60 ms VOTs, also distinguishing these from 20 and 40 ms VOT stimuli. In another experiment he showed that non-speech stimuli (two pure tones with the same temporal relationship) produced very similar evoked potential effects. It therefore seems that the left hemisphere may indeed have specialised in the perceptual analysis of the sort of discriminations which are essential to the understanding of speech.

Evoked potential experiments such as Molfese's have ended up being more informative about process than about localisation of function, and this is their greatest virtue. Even if EEG parameters do vary across hemispheres with stimuli, we have no proof that they reflect processes essential to the one in which we're interested. On the other hand, succeeding in identifying a complex stimulus pattern which is associated with a localised EEG response pattern tells us far more, and is potentially more important, than the mere verification of asymmetry of function.

Asymmetrical Slow Waves

During the 1000 ms before a voluntary response, a negativity develops on the scalp over the motor cortex. It is normally contralaterally asymmetrical, depending on which hand is making the response (McAdam and Seales, 1969). Mapping the 10–20 electrode placement system onto the motor homunculus (see Figure 4.5) shows that left and right hand and finger control lies approximately below positions C3 and C4, respectively, on the surface of the cortex. If any doubt remained that this phenomenon was a product of the sensorimotor cortex, it would be dispelled by the observations of Shibasaki *et al.* (1980) and Brunia and Vingerhoets (1981) that foot responses are preceded by ipsilateral negative slow potentials: the motor cortex responsible for foot movement is actually contralateral, but deep in the central cleft of the cortex, so the left and right dipoles would cross over to the ipsilateral side before being measurable from the scalp. Brunia and Vingerhoets also used a CNV paradigm, with a 4 s ISI, assessing the lateral asymmetry of EEG preceding foot and finger movements, and confirmed their BP findings, that contralateral negativity developed before finger movement rather than before foot movement. Thus, the difference between finger and foot BP only confirmed the well-known cartography of the motor cortex. Observing this phenomenon during the CNV also represents a step closer to resolving the debate about whether the late CNV and the BP are the same component (see Chapter 3).

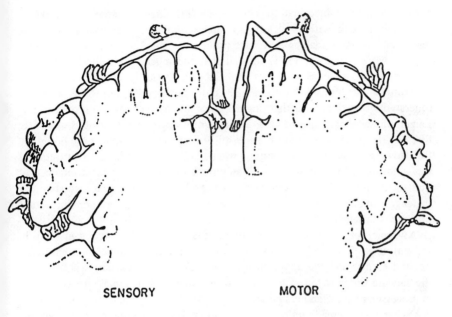

SENSORY   MOTOR

Figure 4.5 The homunculus: the relative representation of different parts of the body over the sensory motor strips of the cortex as revealed by stimulation studies. From Geschwind (1979)

The homunculus shows that face movements originate low down, below temporal positions T3 and T4. Speech involves musculature on both sides of the face, so one might expect the BP to be symmetrical before an utterance. Any asymmetry, with greater negativity over the left side, could therefore be attributed to linguistic rather than motor preparation. Schafer (1967) and McAdam and Whitaker (1973) argued thus when they reported asymmetries in BPs preceding the utterance of polysyllabic words.

Subsequent work showed that these potentials, recorded from T3 and below, were invariably contaminated by movement and respiratory concomitants of preparation for speech. Authors such as Szirtes and Vaughan (1977) and Grozinger *et al.* (1974) left very little room for optimism as to the possibility of separating out any cortical components from the confounded waveforms recorded from these sites. However, Brooker and Donald (1980) have pointed out that the correlation of myogenic events with scalp potentials does not necessarily mean that one caused the other, and that the level of contamination from movement and respiration is relatively slight higher up on the scalp, at locations C3 and C4.

Empson (1982) has argued that it may still be possible to isolate cortical components of the BP preceding vocalisation – in particular, by looking for components which are differentially affected by psychological aspects of speech production. Recording from C3 and C4 to linked mastoids, he found that BPs preceding a repeated word ('yes') were later and smaller than those preceding words which the subject had to generate, going through the alphabet to produce a word beginning with each letter. It appeared that the process of linguistic search and decision-making may have produced a lengthier and larger BP. Subsequent work (Empson, 1983) showed that the repeated production of polysyllabic words, such as the ones that subjects typically emitted in the first experiment, was preceded by large BPs indistinguishable from those preceding generated words. The idea that linguistic search was necessary to produce these longer BPs was obviously wrong, leaving word length as the obvious candidate for the difference — the longer the word to be uttered the longer the preceding BP. However, covariance analysis showed that the actual length of utterances was unimportant in determining BP amplitude 600 ms before the utterance and that the number of syllables in the word was all-important, which suggested that the degree of effort involved in uttering the anticipated word was more important than any other factor.

Asymmetries in BP were noted in the first experiment, but not in the subsequent ones. This series of experiments illustrates the misleading nature of isolated studies and the importance of persistence in establishing what, in fact, the data are trying to tell us. In particular, as in many other studies on asymmetries in processing, the differences between the tasks chosen by the experimenter were not what they seemed, and even when the important parameters distinguishing them have been established, we are left with more questions than answers.

5

Sleep and Dreaming

THE EEG DURING SLEEP

Sleep research has been one of the success stories of EEG. The techniques developed to record and score EEG sleep states have found applications in psychiatry, neurology, animal behaviour and human physiology, as well as in psychology itself. The implications of the findings from EEG studies of sleep have vitally affected theory and research in all these disciplines. Because of the interdisciplinary nature of most of the work on sleep, there will be sections of this chapter which do not directly discuss EEG work but are essential for an understanding of sleep research in general, and of the contribution that electroencephalography has made to it.

Early work by Loomis *et al.* (1936, 1937) in the 1930s established that there were systematic changes in brainwaves with sleep, in that large slow waves developed very soon (within 15 min) after a subject fell asleep at night, and during the night the amplitude of these waves waxed and waned. Loomis established a convention of sleep stages, indicated by the numbers 1 to 6, 6 being the deepest, with the biggest slow waves. Rather puzzlingly, the EEG would sometimes revert to being low-voltage, activated, while the subject was still plainly asleep. These periods of low-voltage sleep were called 'emergent stage 1' because subjects were not as easily roused as from 'ordinary' sleep onset stage 1 sleep, and because, being continuous with deeper stages of sleep, these periods of light sleep were obviously not a transition between wakefulness and sleep, in the way that sleep onset stage 1 seemed to be.

It was not until 1953, when Aserinsky and Kleitman reported rapid, saccadic eye movements, similar in appearance to waking eye movements, associated with periods of low-voltage EEG in both infants and adults, that it became clear that 'emergent stage 1' was indeed a completely different state from 'descending stage 1' — particularly when they also made it clear that the experience of dreaming in adults was almost totally confined to these episodes of 'rapid eye movement' (REM) sleep. In 1961 Ralph Berger (Berger and Oswald, 1962) discovered the loss of tonus in extrinsic laryngeal muscles which accompanies REM sleep. These two findings, linking EEG patterns with eye movement and with neck and throat muscle activity, have formed the basis of the recording and scoring methods for humans now in use all over the world, which have been definitively summarised by Rechtschaffen and Kales (1968). The electromyogram (EMG) and the electro-oculogram (EOG) are both measurable with the standard EEG machine, so that there has been little difficulty in setting up sleep laboratories in hospital EEG departments or in universities. Psychophysiological measures have, in fact, been so enormously successful in the study of sleep that they are now used to define sleep states rather than merely to describe them. Figure 5.1 shows good examples of the psychophysiology associated with relaxed wakefulness and five internationally recognised stages of sleep — four slow wave sleep stages, numbered 1 to 4, and stage REM sleep, which is associated with dreaming. Table 5.1 lists the stages with their defining characteristics.

Table 5.1   Sleep stage scoring criteria

Stage	EEG	EOG	EMG
Awake	Low-voltage, desynchronised. 10 Hz alpha with eyes shut	Saccadic movements, blinks	High tonic level
Stage 1	Low-voltage, desynchronised, No alpha. Some theta bursts or vertex spikes	Slow, rolling eye movements	Moderate tonic level
Stage 2	Low-voltage, desynchronised, with phasic 13–15 Hz spindles and K complexes	EOG dominated by frontal EEG. No eye movements	Moderate tonic level
Stage 3	As stage 2, but increasing slow wave (<2 Hz) activity (20–50% of record)	EOG dominated by frontal EEG. No eye movements	Low tonic level
Stage 4	Slow wave activity increased to >50% of record	EOG dominated by frontal EEG. No eye movements	Low or very low tonic level
Stage REM	Low-voltage, desynchronised, sometimes preceded by 3–7 Hz 'saw-tooth' waves.	Phasic rapid eye movements	Very low tonic level, or non-existent

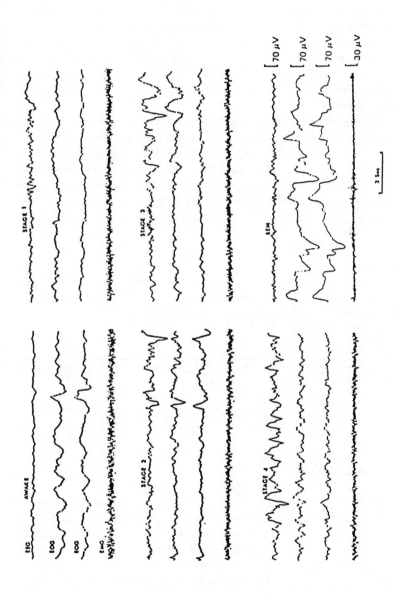

Figure 5.1 Examples of sleep stages as defined by EEG (channel 1), EOG (channels 2 and 3) and submental EMG (channel 4). See Table 5.1 for details of sleep stage scoring criteria

The EEG is used as one of three psychophysiological measures to detect syndromes of activity associated with the different sleep states. So far as slow wave sleep is concerned, the greater the amplitude and period of the EEG slow waves the deeper the sleep, and EMG and EOG changes are largely irrelevant. These only become crucial in discriminating REM sleep from stage 1 sleep (when the rapid eye movements in the EOG and the loss of muscle tone in the EMG indicate REM sleep), and stage 1 sleep from relaxed wakefulness (when the slow, rolling eye movements of stage 1 are easily distinguished from the rapid eye movements of REM, and the level of muscle tone is, again, a definitive sign of stage REM sleep).

Figure 5.2 shows the typical patterning of sleep through the night, as shown by a healthy adult. On going to sleep, all normal people start with slow wave sleep, and do not have any REM sleep until at least 45 min have elapsed. There is then an alternation between slow wave sleep and REM sleep, with REM sleep recurring about every 90 min. The first REM sleep period is usually shorter than the subsequent ones — about 15 min in adults, as against later periods of about 30 min. Deep slow wave sleep (stage 4) predominates in the first half of the night.

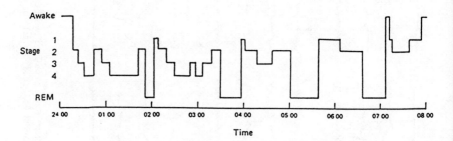

Figure 5.2   A typical night's sleep for a young adult

SLEEPING BEHAVIOUR

Sleepers can easily be woken up, so it is obvious that attentional and perceptual processes are functioning at some level. Oswald *et al.* (1960) took advantage of the fact that during stage 2 sleep it is commonplace to elicit very large EEG potentials ('K complexes') of about 150 μV from peak to trough with quite quiet sounds. (K complexes also occur spontaneously, with no stimulation.) They instructed their subjects to listen out for particular names, and then played a variety of names to them, including their own. The K complex responses to the target names were larger and more reliable than to control names, and subjects also almost invariably responded to their own name with a large K complex — another example of the so-called 'cocktail party effect', where one unerringly picks out fragments of conversation relating to oneself from a medley of sounds. An experiment reported by Langford *et al.* (1974) which showed that awakening latency was faster to a subject's own name played forwards than backwards confirmed this finding. Anecdotal evidence of being able to listen out for babies' cries, or other particular sounds, are, of course, very commonplace. Not surprisingly, the empirical evidence confirms this ubiquitous experience. This behaviour could be supported by attentional mechanisms of a simple template matching sort (that we are familiar with in the orienting response) rather than the more complex processing that goes on during wakefulness.

McDonald *et al.* (1975) repeated the Oswald group's experiment, also finding that K complexes were more reliably elicited by a subject's own name than by somebody else's, and showing that this effect was measurable in heart rate (HR) and finger plethysmograph (FP – measuring the blood supply to the skin, which is normally reduced by alerting or alarming stimuli). While the overwhelmingly large EEG slow waves of stages 3 and 4 make it impracticable to record K complexes, the McDonald group were able to show, using these other measures, that perceptual discriminations were also being made in stage REM sleep, although not in stages 3 and 4.

In another experiment, the subjects were conditioned while awake to associate a highly unpleasant blast of noise (produced by 'two pairs of dual freon boat horns') with either a low-pitch or a high-pitch tone of relatively low intensity (40 dB). The conditioned signal elicited FP and HR responses in all stages of slow wave sleep, including stages 3 and 4, and K complexes in stage 2. Interestingly, these conditioned stimuli (undoubtedly well-established, since responses were made to them in the other sleep stages) did not produce any response in REM sleep. Since it is well established that meaningful stimuli can be processed and responded to during REM sleep, the authors argued that these findings support the notion that only cognitively meaningful material is dealt with in this sleep stage. They could also be interpreted as evidence for REM sleep mentation being peculiarly efficient at coping with stimuli denoting unpleasant consequences. This is, in essence, the Freudian view of what 'dreamwork' does – render potentially upsetting internally generated ideas harmless by transforming them into symbolic codes.

However, neither of these studies throws much light on the actual level of perceptual processing going on, since only *particular* stimuli, previously defined during wakefulness, were used. Subjects did not have to do more than set up 'templates' to recognise these particular sounds.

Sleep Learning

One of the earliest applications of the EEG in assessing perceptual and memory functioning during sleep was directed at 'sleep learning' – the rather attractive notion that instead of the student having to work away learning material during the day, it could be painlessly absorbed while the student was fast asleep. In order to test this idea, Emmons and Simon in 1956 used EEG recordings to present material *only* when subjects were indubitably asleep. Subjects showed no recollection next day of this material presented to them during sleep. However, there is evidence that fairly subtle perceptual processing can go on during sleep. Evans *et al.* (1970) made verbal suggestions to sleeping subjects that their left or right leg would become cramped and uncomfortable when they heard a particular word. Subjects moved the appropriate leg as though it were indeed uncomfortable. This 'sleep learning' was retained very well over a week, and one of the subjects tested asleep again after 6 months still moved the leg when given the word learned when asleep 6 months earlier. No recollection of these cue words could be elicited from the subjects during the day, either by direct questioning or by use of indirect free associative techniques.

This result intriguingly suggests a dissociation between waking and sleeping life, reminding one of the dilemma of Chuang-tzu, the Chinese philosopher, who posed the following in the third century B.C.: 'One night I dreamed that I was a butterfly, fluttering hither and thither, content with my lot. Suddenly, I awoke and I was Chuang-tzu again. Who am I in reality? A butterfly dreaming that I am Chuang-tzu or Chuang-tzu imagining he was a butterfly?'.

To return to the issue of whether learning can take place during a sleep period, one might ask whether stimuli which woke the subject up would be remembered. Portnoff *et al.* (1966) woke subjects up throughout the night and presented them with lists of words to remember. They were then either allowed to go back to sleep immediately or kept awake for 5 min. Next day the subjects could not recall very many of the words they had seen when they had been allowed to go back to sleep immediately, and recalled many more from the trials after which they had been kept awake for a while, although they had shown just as much evidence of learning in both conditions. Similarly, Koukkou and Lehmann (1968) found that sentences read out to sleeping subjects were not recalled next day unless the subjects had both been woken by the presentation and stayed awake (with measurable alpha in EEG) for at least 2 min. Taken together, these experiments suggest that the immediate consolidation of memory is prevented by sleep, or disrupted by going to sleep.

DREAMING

Incorporation of Stimuli into Dreams, and Dreamwork

Almost everybody has a story to tell about dream incorporation – for instance, dreaming about Arctic exploration only to wake up and find that the covers have slipped off and they're freezing cold, or dreaming of bells ringing only to wake up eventually to find that the alarm clock has been clattering for the last few minutes. Are these dreams really triggered by outside stimuli or are these reports only the outcome of rather memorable coincidences? Dement and Wolpert (1958) verified that external stimuli could indeed be incorporated into dreams during REM sleep. An example they gave is: 'The S was sleeping on his stomach. His back was uncovered. An eye movement period started and after it had persisted for 10 minutes, cold water was sprayed on his back. Exactly 30 seconds later he was awakened. The first part of the dream involved a rather complex description of acting in a play. Then, "I was walking behind the leading lady when she suddenly collapsed and water was dripping on her face. I ran over to her and felt water dripping on my back and head. The roof was leaking. I was very puzzled why she fell down and decided some plaster must have fallen on her. I looked up and there was a hole in the roof. I dragged her over to the side of the stage and began pulling the curtains. Just then I woke up." '

Dement (1974) reports some further experiments in his book *Some Must Watch While Some Must Sleep*. (This book also includes fascinating anecdotes about the background to most of the pioneering experiments of the 1960s: Dement was personally involved in many of them.) Using a variety of sound stimuli, such as bugles, Dement and his students started the tape recordings as soon as an REM period started. They found that the dreams reported by the subjects were noticeably affected by the stimuli on over half of the occasions. The incorporation of stimuli is thus extremely common, if not invariable (given that on many occasions the effects of stimulation on dreaming will be so idio-syncratic that they are not recognised by experimenters).

The orthodox psychoanalytic view of the processes underlying dream incorporation is that they maintain sleep. That is, internally generated ideas which would otherwise cause the subject to wake up blushing with shame or racked with guilt are transformed by the dreamwork into a symbolic code. In the same way, external stimuli become incorporated into dreams in order to reduce their arousing effect. The experimental evidence does not contradict this view, but neither does it support it very strongly. The notion of dreamwork involves an assumption about the function of dreaming (and possibly of consciousness in general) – i.e. that the dream is controlling the subject's psychological state, and not the other way around. That is, it could be that stimuli which fail to arouse the brain sufficiently to tip it into wakefulness result in dream incorporation rather than that the dream incorporation results in continued sleeping. Experimental evidence (Bradley and Meddis, 1974) shows that the incorporation of stimuli into dreaming is indeed associated with continued sleep rather than with wakening. Whether the incorporation actually protects sleep, as the Freudian theory would predict, or whether incorporation is the consequence of delayed arousal remains unclear.

Internally generated stimuli (such as feelings of hunger or thirst) do not seem to have a simple effect on dream content. Again, Freudian theory might seem to have a straightforward prediction, that the process of wish-fulfilment would inevitably cause thirsty subjects to dream of quenching their thirst, hungry

subjects to dream of eating. Volunteers in an experiment on the effects of pro-
longed starvation conducted by Ancel Keys in the 1940s did not report an
increase in dreams about food (Keys *et al.*, 1950). Dement and Wolpert (1958)
worked on the effects of thirst on dreaming in the laboratory, obtaining REM-
awakening reports from volunteers who had not had any fluid intake for at least
24 h. They recorded not one instance of drinking or of thirst in a dream. They
did record five instances of dreams which were clearly related to the theme of
drinking and thirst, although not explicitly so. The so-called dreamwork, which
(in Freudian theory) disguises unacceptable ideas as the manifest dream, could
be interpreted as having been involved here. But why should thirst be counted as
an unacceptable idea? Possibly the transformation of ideas in dreaming takes
place regardless of its emotional connotations. However, people who give up
smoking very frequently have explicit dreams about smoking in the first few
weeks of withdrawal — possibly confirming the notion of wish-fulfilment, but
not consistent with the idea of invariable dreamwork.

Presleep Stimulation and Dreaming

It is very well known that dreams often contain elements — visual or ideational
— that can be identified as being part of the previous day's experience. Much of
our dream content is not so easily traced, but the incorporation of 'day's residues'
into dreams is very well established. In a systematic study of his own dream-life,
Freud tried to relate all his dreams to feelings and thoughts experienced the
previous day. It was not possible to do this without assuming that dreamwork
transformations took place. That is, the 'manifest dream's' apparently irrelevant
and unpredictable content was actually deemed to have been systematically
arrived at from a 'latent dream', whose implicit content had been the subject of
some extensive dreamwork. Therefore, with sufficient ingenuity, an analyst can
trace any reported dream back to certain themes which he or she believes are
preoccupying the dreamer. If we could be sure that all dream content is determined in this way, then this would not be an unreasonable thing to do.

Experimental studies relating presleep stimulation to dream content are not
obviously encouraging in this respect. Foulkes and Rechtschaffen (1964) showed
either an amusing or a violent TV Western to subjects before bed-time, and found
that although the violent film reliably induced more vivid, emotional dreams,
direct incorporation of the content of either film was very rare indeed.
Goodenough *et al.* (1975) confirmed that the emotional content of dreams
could be affected by presleep stimulation (in this case, a film entitled *Subcision*
— explicitly showing a series of operations carried out on the penis as part of a
tribal aboriginal initiation rite).

The fact that upsetting or emotionally significant events are not directly
incorporated into dreams does not, of course, disprove any psychoanalytic theory
of the origin and function of dreaming. In fact, paradoxically, one could argue

that it offers the idea of dreamwork some support, and that the manifest dreams only need the appropriate analysis to reveal that the latent dreams are full of references to this material. Scientifically speaking, we are still at the stage of describing the natural history of dreams, and have no solid ground for ascribing functions to them. However, this has not prevented a number of theories from being put forward – in particular, relating dreaming to some aspect of computer functioning. Evans and Newman (1964) suggested that dreaming was analogous to 'off-line processing' – i.e. that a back-log of intellectual activity built up during the day, which could be caught up with during sleep, and also that new ideas (analogous to the development of new programming systems in the computer) could be tried out in dreaming which might otherwise be too risky to attempt during wakefulness.

More recently, Crick and Mitchison (1983) have suggested that dreams are the only demonstrable outcome of a brain mechanism whose function is the unlearning of useless connections in the brain, the forgetting of redundant information. Computer simulations by Hopfield *et al.* (1983) suggested that the random stimulation of a complex system could regularly resolve into a small number of stereotyped outcomes. During dreaming sleep, the cortex is being bombarded with stimulation from the hindbrain, which, according to Crick and Mitchison, results in the experience of dreaming (with its frequently repetitive symbolic code) as a by-product of unlearning. This theory is a subtle combination of neurophysiology, computer technology and psychology, and has not yet been tested. One comment that may be pertinent is that 'unlearning' in the literal sense that is meant in neurophysiology may even result in consolidation and sharpening of memories rather than simply in forgetting, in that everything we know about the psychology of memory suggests that it is the organisation of memories that is crucially important in determining the memorability of individual events, and not the 'strength' of individual memory 'traces'.

A common assumption is that we somehow ought to have an explanation of the nature of dreaming consciousness, although few would maintain that we have a firm idea of the nature or function of 'normal', waking consciousness. A recurring theme in the theoretical treatment of dreaming is that dreams are bizarre and imaginative compared with waking consciousness. Rechtschaffen (1978) challenged this notion, in one of the very few systematic comparisons of dreaming with waking consciousness. During normal consciousness, he argued, there are often two streams of thought – one containing 'voluntary' mental productions, which may be relatively task-oriented, and the other being a reflective process, apparently monitoring and commenting on the first. During dreaming, the second stream is absent, and, most important, it is, he claimed, not possible for the second stream of consciousness to imagine. When awake it would be unremarkable to claim to be imagining an outdoor scene when sitting at one's desk. If dreaming of sitting at a desk, Rechtschaffen claimed, it is not possible to imagine anything else. Dreams are thus non-reflective (what he called 'single-minded') and non-imaginative. This is not to say that they are not organised creations, and Rechtschaffen also points out that the freedom from preconceived notions that the non-reflective style of consciousness provides may be essential to the creativity of dreaming.

THE RHYTHMS OF SLEEP

This section will deal with effects of various regimens on sleep, both throwing light on sleep mechanisms and providing clues as to the function of sleep. A great advantage of sleep research is the unselfconsciousness of the sleeping subject. It is normally very difficult to observe spontaneous behaviour in adults without the mere presence of the observer strongly affecting what is observed. When sleep mechanisms take over, there is little scope for selfconsciousness. Psychophysiological recordings then allow of direct measurement of the sleeping brain's free-running rhythms, or its response to experimental manipulation, including, for instance, deprivation of food and sleep itself, or the effects of exercise.

Food and Sleep

People will frequently ascribe the quality of sleep (or lack of it) to the previous night's food intake. It is undoubtedly true that indigestion will disturb sleep, but does food have any more subtle effects? Brezinova and Oswald (1972) set out to test the efficacy of Horlicks as a night-time drink, intended to induce sleep, using a young adult group (mean age 22 years) and an older group (mean age 55 years). They found that while Horlicks (or, in fact, another malted milk drink) had little effect on sleep onset time in either group, restlessness during the night was reduced in both, and in the older subjects the advantage conferred by the nourishing bed-time drinks was greatest in the second half of the night, reducing restlessness and increasing total sleep time.

Drastic reductions in food intake are symptomatic of anorexia nervosa, and patients suffering from this condition were found by Crisp and Stonehill (1977) to sleep little and fitfully. When the same people were putting on weight, they slept more, and with fewer interruptions. Also, there was a change in the proportion of different stages of sleep during remission, so that there was a massive increase in the amount of deep slow wave sleep at the expense of light slow wave sleep stages. These findings are consistent with the idea that slow wave sleep is concerned with bodily anabolic processes, which will be discussed more fully later in the chapter.

Exercise and Sleep

As with food, folklore has much to say about exercise and its effects on sleep — to claim a good night's sleep to be the result of strenuous exercise the previous day is entirely uncontroversial. However, the experimental evidence on the subject is by no means unambiguous. Baekeland and Laski (1966), Hauri (1966) and Zir *et al.* (1971) found that human sleep was unaffected by large amounts of exercise the previous day, although evidence from experiments on rats had shown that prolonged exercise increased the amount of slow wave sleep.

Comparing the effects of exercise in trained and untrained subjects, Walker *et al.* (1978) found no effect of exercise, while Griffin and Trinder (1978) reported an increase in slow wave (stage 3) sleep in the trained subjects. Horne and Porter (1976) also found an increase in stage 3 sleep in the first half of the night, following exercise. The large number of studies addressing themselves to this issue have varied considerably in the amount of exercise used, the physical fitness of the subjects, the length of time over which they were monitored and the scoring system for slow wave sleep. From a comprehensive review of the evidence, Horne (1981) concluded that untrained subjects show little if any sleep EEG effects following day-time exercise, while trained subjects do have increases in stages 3 and 4 in the first recovery night after raised exercise *rate*. That is, the deep slow wave sleep stages are elevated if the rate of energy expenditure during the day is increased, rather than merely the total amount.

Bunnell *et al.* (1983) followed up this suggestion with an experiment in which subjects' rate of energy expenditure (REE) was elevated to a high level, but not for long enough to significantly affect the total energy expenditure (TEE) for the day. The increase in stages 3 and 4 sleep before the first REM sleep period of the night was of the same order as had been found in other experiments when both REE and TEE had been increased. The idea that exercise might increase the need for bodily restitution through its heavy energy demands, and that deep slow wave sleep would then be increased to accommodate this requirement, is unsupported by this evidence. Rather, the effects are probably mediated through some other change caused by exercise, such as increased body temperature.

Horne and Moore (1985) showed that athletes who exercised strenuously in their track-suits, with no cooling, showed elevations in rectal temperature of over 2°C, and elevated levels of stage 4 sleep the following night. When exercised in light, damp clothing, under cooling fans, the same athletes showed an increase of rectal temperature of only 1°C and no change in sleep from baseline levels. Similarly, Horne and Reid (1985) have shown that passive heating (by lying in a warm bath for 90 min) also caused increases in stage 4 sleep. Body temperature clearly affects sleep, and later in this chapter a study on crocodiles will be described which showed that warming the animals produced evidence of slow waves in the sleeping EEG which had not hitherto been observed in reptiles. Since the total amount of exercise expended does not determine sleep quality so much as the rate achieved, it is unlikely that this effect is mediated through the effect on metabolic rate over the day. It is unclear as yet whether the changes in human sleep are caused by the effects of warming on the musculature or whether brain temperature itself can be altered by these procedures, and affect the quality of sleep directly.

Effects of Sleep Deprivation on Subsequent Sleep

It is a commonplace observation that if we lose a night's sleep, we tend to sleep rather longer on subsequent nights, as if to make up a 'sleep debt'. Generally speaking, the amount of sleep lost is not made up for entirely on the recovery nights. Recordings of the EEG of recovery sleep have shown that the first night is characterised by a great increase in stage 4 sleep, at the expense of the lighter slow wave sleep stages (Berger and Oswald, 1962). During the second and sub-sequent recovery nights, subjects typically show a relative elevation of REM sleep levels (Kales *et al.*, 1970). Thus, stage 4 and REM sleep are almost made up, while stage 2 sleep is not. Like the evidence from the partial deprivation experiments (and, incidentally, from neurophysiological evidence beyond the scope of this book), these data suggest that the two main sleep states have distinct control mechanisms.

Effects of Partial Deprivation on Subsequent Sleep

Since normal subjects *always* begin a sleep period with slow wave sleep, only periodically returning to REM sleep, it was naturally asked what would happen if they were woken whenever they attempted to start an REM sleep period. When allowed to return to sleep, would they pick up where they left off, starting REM sleep, or would they start the night all over again? Dement (1960) woke six subjects in this systematic way over a period of six nights, and found that on the first night they did seem to 'start all over again' whenever properly woken, so that by the end of the night they had achieved a good deal of slow wave sleep and very little REM sleep. On subsequent nights it became more difficult to prevent REM sleep, especially in the early hours, and the number of wakenings necessary increased night by night until, by the fifth and sixth nights, subjects were getting hardly any sleep at all. There is thus a distinct drive for REM sleep. On recovery nights, when subjects were allowed to sleep undisturbed, they took more REM sleep than usual, as if they were making up to some extent for the amount lost.

    Like REM sleep, stage 4 sleep is 'fragile' in the sense that systematic disruption can cause its replacement by light slow wave sleep (stages 1 and 2). Agnew *et al.* (1964) showed that there is also a specific rebound phenomenon on recovery nights, so that up to 50 per cent of stage 4 sleep 'lost' is made up.

Sleep Stage Cycling and Circadian Entrainment

Many physiological processes are organised on a daily basis. Thus, body tem-perature falls during the evening to a minimum in the early hours, independently of activity. Similarly, blood and urine constituents vary systematically over the

24 hours, reflecting circadian variations in metabolism. During a typical night's sleep the deep slow wave stages predominate in the first two or three hours, and light slow wave sleep, alternating with relatively long periods of REM sleep, is characteristic during the second half of the night.

Webb and Agnew (1964) and Hume and Mill (1977) have shown that while stage 4 sleep can occur at any time of the day or night, always appearing early in a sleep period whenever it starts, REM sleep periods are short and relatively unstable at all hours of the day, apart from the early hours of the morning.

Studies of the sleep of shift-workers have shown that they suffer from disturbed sleep during the day and that REM sleep, in particular, suffers a severe reduction when a worker is sleeping during the day (see, e.g., Tilley and Wilkinson, 1982). It loses out in competition with stage 4 at the beginning of the sleep period, in the morning, and then the drive for REM appears to dissipate later in the sleep period, during the early afternoon.

The Ninety-minute Cycle – Does It Run All Day?

The alternation between slow wave sleep and REM sleep during the night was described by Kleitman (1969) as the expression of a phylogenetically old basic rest–activity cycle (BRAC), which, he suggested, continued during the day, and on which the sleep-wakefulness cycle was superimposed. An alternative explanation is that the cycling is the outcome of a homeostatic interplay between mechanisms controlling REM and non-REM sleep. Ephron and Carrington (1966) were among the first to suggest this, explaining that the periodic REM sleep phases could be a method of maintaining arousal in an otherwise increasingly unresponsive brain. If this were true, we would expect the timing and quantity of REM sleep to be determined principally by the amount and depth of prior slow wave sleep. This does not appear to be the case. In fact, there is evidence (Globus *et al.*, 1969) that the timing of REM sleep periods is to some extent 'preprogrammed', so that they occur at the same times of night, regardless of when the subjects went to sleep or whether they 'missed' an REM period. While the entrainment of 90 min cycles into the 24 h day has not always been observed in subsequent studies, Globus's work stimulated the study of periodicity during the day, as well as the study of sleeping cycles.

Carskadon and Dement (1975) reported an elegant and ingenious experiment which resolved the question of whether sleep mechanisms for the main sleep states were interdependent in this way. Their five subjects followed a regimen of a succession of 90 min 'days' for almost a week, being allowed sleep for 30 min periods with waking intervals of 60 min. If the Ephron and Carrington model were right, the subjects should never develop any REM sleep, since slow wave sleep could not 'accumulate'. In the event, all the subjects showed all the normal sleep stages, but frequently went straight from waking to stage REM sleep (REM sleep occurred within 10 min of sleep onset in 79 out of the 110 sleep periods containing REM sleep). They typically alternated the type of sleep between successive sleep periods, although REM sleep was primarily between 07.30 and 14.00.

Sleep mechanisms are therefore normally entrained to their own endogenous clock with a period of about 90 min, which may itself be entrained to the ubiquitous circadian cycle. It follows from this that the 90 min clock is also ticking over during the day (and some of Globus's work on the timing of REM sleep periods during afternoon naps supports this idea). If so, does it affect waking behaviour? Friedman and Fisher (1967) observed a group of psychiatric patients over periods of 6 h, and counted the number and timing of eating, drinking and other oral behaviours. Deeply committed to Freudian theory, they devised a scoring system which, for instance, gave 10 points for a drink of milk (because of its symbolic importance) and only 1 point for a sandwich. A clear 90 min cycle in oral behaviour was evident, which they interpreted as being a manifestation of the sublimated outcome of fluctuations in erotic drive level.

The Friedman and Fisher experiment suffers from two major flaws. First, subjects were observed as a group, so that interactions between the patients may have led to their eating and drinking cyclically at the same time. Second, the food and drink available was nutritious, and thus certainly directly affected their level of appetite: the study becomes much less interesting if the results merely reflected the timing of gastrointestinal processes. Oswald *et al.* (1970) repeated the experiment, using non-nutritive foods and drink, and with their six subjects isolated from one another. A simple count of the timing of feeding and drinking (with no complicated points system) confirmed that there was a 90 min cycle (see Figure 5.3).

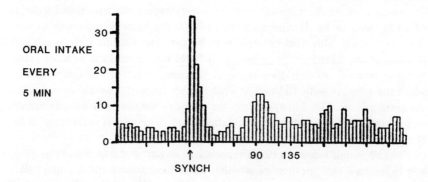

Figure 5.3 Distribution of oral intake scores when peak intakes were synchronised for the period from 0 h 30 min to 2 h from the start. From Oswald *et al.* (1970)

If the BRAC (basic rest–activity cycle) persists during the day, how does it affect cognitive processing and performance? Klein and Armitage (1979) reasoned that since there is evidence for relative activation of the right hemisphere during

REM sleep with respect to the left, the times of day which would contain REM sleep, were the subject asleep, should also be characterised by right hemisphere activation, which would result in improved performance on tasks tapping spatial abilities and worse performance on tasks tapping verbal abilities. They tested eight subjects over a period of 8 h, using verbal and spatial tasks, and found that performance on both showed evidence of periodicity with a peak of 96 min. What is more, these cycles in efficiency were 180 degrees out of phase, just as they had predicted. If the two sides of the brain indeed become activated on a 90 min cycle, then this should be reflected in power in the EEG. Manseau and Broughton (1984) confirmed that there is a significant cycling in EEG power, at 72–120 min period, during a day of isolation in their eight subjects, but did not find any difference between the hemispheres, recording from F3, F4, P3 and P4. They suggested that the brainstem reticular activating system may be responsible for this cycling in arousal level rather than any mechanisms intrinsic to the cerebral hemispheres.

While these experiments have provided good evidence for 90 min periodicity in day-time behaviour, and it is reasonable to assume that this is related to the sleeping 90 min cycle, it remains to be positively demonstrated that day-time fluctuations in performance are determined by the REM–non-REM sleep cycle of the previous night.

THE EVOLUTION, DEVELOPMENT AND FUNCTIONS OF SLEEP

As the evidence discussed so far has shown, sleep is an unusually stereotyped activity, both behaviourally and physiologically. Almost every human being goes through the same rough pattern of electrophysiological changes every night of the year. Although predictably affected by age and to some extent by drugs, diet and exercise, sleep still seems a largely autonomous process relatively impervious to the vicissitudes of life. The parallel to processes essential to metabolism, such as respiration and digestion, is obvious. The difference is that we understand the role these play in metabolism, as well as the mechanisms, or drives, regulating breathing, eating and drinking, while the functions of sleep remain mysterious. EEG evidence has been critical in the description of sleep as well as in the investigation of the drives regulating sleep states, especially in deprivation experiments. In order to establish the physiological function of a process like this, however, it becomes necessary to understand its role in fulfilling physiological needs, which may not always be obvious, and which may be somewhat obscurely related to drive mechanisms. Breathing, for instance, provides a supply of oxygen essential for metabolism. The drive mechanism regulating the ventilation of the lungs is unaffected by oxygen levels in the blood, but is very sensitive indeed to the acidity of the blood — normally determined by carbon dioxide dissolved as carbonic acid. The rather more subtle functions of sleep will probably be suggested even more obliquely by their drive mechanisms than those driving respiration.

Table 5.2 shows norms for sleep parameters over a range of ages. These data have been derived from the percentages given by Williams *et al.* (1974), and are based on about twenty subjects in each age group. They confirm the general findings of previous studies, based on fewer subjects (see, e.g., Roffwarg *et al.*, 1966; Feinberg, 1968).

Table 5.2 Sleep achieved in the laboratory by subjects of different ages. From Williams *et al.* (1974)

Age group	Total sleep time (min/night)	Sleep latency	Sleep stages 1	2	3	4	REM	Wakenings	Number of subjects
3–5	594	14	12	276	18	102	186	1	21
6–9	581	12	12	280	17	99	163	1	22
10–12	560	17	17	267	23	97	153	1	24
13–15	484	16	20	230	25	83	127	3	20
16–19	451	18	18	224	27	78	101	2	23
20–29	425	14	17	205	26	60	116	2	21
30–39	424	8	22	237	26	30	108	2	20
40–49	407	9	29	278	25	13	106	4	21
50–59	410	11	25	250	21	13	93	5	23
60–69	406	13	40	243	13	8	97	6	21
70–79	393	24	41	248	14	9	92	7	21

The youngest subjects (3-5-year-olds) took about 10 h sleep, compared with the adults' 7, and the additional 3 h was made up almost entirely of REM sleep (twice as much) and stage 4 (50 per cent more than in adults). Theories relating sleep functions to anabolic processes and growth (Roffwarg *et al.*, 1966; Oswald, 1969) have relied heavily on this evidence for increased levels of sleep being correlated with the periods of maximum growth. REM sleep quantity seems to be well correlated with brain weight increase in the early years, and Oswald (1969) hypothesised that brain protein synthesis is elevated during REM sleep.

Oswald's empirical contribution was concerned with the time course of recovery of normal sleep after drug overdoses and drug withdrawal, and other brain insults such as intensive ECT. He found that all these traumatic insults to the central nervous system were followed, in the patients who survived, by pro-longed elevations in the quantity of REM sleep. The time scales involved are also very consistent with estimated times for the half-life of amino acids in the brain. (While brain nerve cells are not replaced if they die, there is a constant turnover of protein in brain tissue, so that in a 6 week period about half the total protein in the brain is replaced.) He suggested that the increases in REM sleep time which occur after drug withdrawal or drug overdose are a manifestation of recovery processes going on in the brain, involving intensive neuronal protein synthesis. High amounts of REM sleep in the very young are thus a consequence of brain growth, and adult anabolic and recovery processes in the brain are similarly seen to require REM sleep.

Stage 4 sleep does not develop until about 6 months post-partum, but then and thereafter the quantity taken is well correlated with bodily growth in the juvenile. The nocturnal secretion of growth hormone (which stimulates somatic protein synthesis in the growing animal) is actually dependent on uninterrupted stage 4 sleep (Sassin *et al.*, 1969). In adulthood a chronic lack of normal stage 4 sleep is found in sufferers from fibrositis, whose EEG during deep sleep is characterised by 'alpha–delta' patterns — a mixture of sleeping and waking EEG which typically results in the experience of fitful, 'unrestorative' sleep, leaving the patient feeling as tired next day as he or she did before going to bed. (See Chapter 6 for more details of the syndrome of alpha–delta sleep.) Not only do these patients show aberrations in stage 4 sleep, but also the disturbance of stage 4 sleep in healthy volunteers actually causes the symptoms of fibrositis to appear (Muldofsky *et al.*, 1975). All this evidence is consistent with a general anabolic function for sleep: REM sleep subserving brain growth, repair and memory functions, and slow wave (stage 4) sleep promoting bodily growth and repair.

This theory implies that memory processes will be affected by the amount of REM sleep during the night, since it is indisputable that the consolidation of memories will involve protein changes of some sort in the brain. Empson and Clarke (1970) set out to test this hypothesis directly, depriving subjects of REM sleep and measuring the effects of the regimen on the retention of material learned the day before. Ten pairs of yoked subjects were used, who had learned the same materials the evening before, and were both woken up whenever the experimental subject was roused from REM sleep. They found that the retention of complex material (stories) was greatly reduced by REM deprivation, while the retention of lists of words was not. The retention of syntactically correct but meaningless sentences suffered an intermediate amount. Fowler *et al.* (1973) and others have confirmed that REM sleep deprivation has little effect on the retention of meaningless material. Following up on this work, Tilley and Empson (1978) showed that REM sleep deprivation is also more disruptive of memory consolidation in human subjects than stage 4 sleep deprivation, so it is unlikely that the effects observed were non-specific consequences of a stressful regimen. In this context, a fascinating study of 3-month-old babies by Fagen and Rovee-Collier (1983) showed that babies who had apparently forgotten about a kickable overhead mobile and were reminded of its existence showed reminiscence (improved evidence of memory retention) in proportion to the amount of sleep intervening between the reminder and the test. Of course, there is no direct evidence that REM sleep was implicated, but it is very tempting to speculate, given that babies' quiet sleep is largely REM, that the reactivation of old memories could be a function of REM sleep, as much as the consolidation of new ones.

This account of sleep function, the Oswald theory, is an expression of what many non-specialists would subscribe to as being a common-sense view of sleep being good for you, especially in growing children. While the theory is supported by a good deal of evidence, it is all, so to speak, correlational — there is no con-clusive evidence linking sleep with restorative processes. The correlation of periods of growth in the young with high levels of REM sleep could, of course, be fortuitous, and need not indicate that REM sleep is essential to growth. Indeed, the theory has already required some revision. Adam (1980), for instance, pointed out that in some small - mammals the time required protein synthesis is too long to allow for the completion of significant amounts during their short REM periods, so that if REM sleep has any particular significance for brain protein synthesis in these animals, it must be in influencing the quality of protein production rather than simply accelerating the rate. Recent behavioural evidence (Empson *et al.*, 1981) suggests that the advantage given retention of memories by REM sleep relies on an orderly sequence of REM sleep periods, in that the beneficial effect of REM sleep later in the night seemed to be dependent on the uninterrupted completion of a short period of REM sleep early in the night. If true, could this be subserved by slow processes involving protein synthesis, initiated early in the night and continued periodically in REM sleep periods throughout the night? Comparing the brain to an automatic washing machine might be an oversimplification as a general model, but it seems a useful metaphor to explain this sort of cyclical, programmed process.

Is Sleep a Waste of Time?

This is, in fact, a worth-while question to ask. During the early 1970s the common-sense theories of restorative sleep were becoming enshrined as scientific fact long before they had been proven, when a few quiet voices started to question their whole basis. The most fully developed expression of this point of view has been presented by Meddis (1977, 1983), arguing that sleep is a period of enforced inactivity, reducing metabolic demands and keeping the organism out of trouble during periods of the day when other essential needs have been satisfied. Accord-ing to this view, sleep mechanisms evolved in the same way as other instincts — for instance, those controlling the courtship and mating of birds and fish. This provocative theory graphically illustrates the weakness of the evidence supporting the restorative theories, in that it cannot be dismissed out of hand, and a thorough reconsideration of all the assumptions underlying our thinking about sleep function is required to meet its arguments. If this is all the theory has achieved, it will have done a great service.

Obviously, sleep mechanisms must have evolved, and any theory has to explain the variety of life-style across species, involving very great differences in total sleep time in modern species in terms of evolution. If we take the 'waste of time' proposition seriously, it becomes difficult to explain why this particular instinct has become a universal, while other instincts are as diverse as the habitats of the creatures exhibiting them. In particular, it has to explain how this particular instinct remains as a determinant of stereotyped behaviour in mammals when the role of learning has become crucial in the expression of all other mammalian instincts. Nor can it explain why every known mammal shows the same patterning of sleep (although there is great variation in the total quantity taken). Despite enormous differences in life-style, all mammals seem to have to find time for a minimum amount of sleep. Thus, the porpoise has even evolved a system of sleeping with the two sides of the brain alternately (Mukhametov and Poliakove, 1981). If there were no other evidence for the absolute necessity of sleep, this would be eloquent enough on its own. This clearly suggests that sleep has acquired an essential role in physiology, whatever the evolutionary pressures which led to its appearance in primeval reptiles.

A more critical test of the essential nature of sleep is to consider the effects of sleep deprivation. Preventing the expression of some instincts (such as by crowding chickens in small cages) does not result in death, but may produce faster growth and egg-laying. However, interfering with sleep is a much more serious matter (Manaceine, 1897): 'Direct experiment has shown that animals entirely deprived of food for twenty days, and which have then lost more than half their weight, may yet escape death if fed with precaution — that is to say, in small amounts often repeated. On the other hand, I found by experimenting on ten puppies that the complete deprivation of sleep for four or five days (96 to 120 hours) causes irreparable lesions in the organism, and in spite of every care the subjects of these experiments could not be saved. Complete absence of sleep during this period is fatal to puppies in spite of the food taken during this time, and the younger the puppy the more quickly he succumbed.'

With an experiment like this, it is crucially important to know how much physical ill-treatment the dogs were subjected to, to ensure wakefulness, and Manaceine wrote little to reassure one in this respect. Early American work on rats (by Patrick and Gilbert, 1896) involved keeping the animals awake by revolving them in cages. All died from bites inflicted on one another, and, of course, little can be said about the role of sleep from results like that! The puppy experiment was repeated by Kleitman (1927), using 12 animals, which were deprived of sleep for 2–7 days. Unlike Manaceine, Kleitman gives full details of the methods he used to enforce wakefulness, stressing the importance he attached to avoiding any physical damage being inflicted on his dogs. A slight pull on the chain and a short walk would result in wakefulness persisting for some time. Control puppies (allowed unlimited sleep) were introduced to play with the experimental puppies, and this often banished somnolence entirely. Despite this relatively gentle regimen two of the puppies died, and, like Manaceine's dogs, all showed a marked drop in red blood cells.

Oswald (1980) describes how the hormone patterns during wakefulness promote catabolism, while sleep seems necessary for the pattern promoting anabolic processes at night. The impulse to ascribe a functional role to sleep will obviously not be satisfied until we have a clearer understanding of the interactions of the slow neurophysiological swings which punctuate our circadian cycle. To know that sleep deprivation kills is not to know for certain that sleep is restorative in function — it is vital to understand the mechanisms involved as well. The contention that sleep serves no function has been useful in forcing a critical re-examination of our sometimes unwarranted preconceptions and assumptions about the role of sleep. The Oswald theory has been particularly useful in the role that theory must have, of tying facts into bundles — almost everything we know about sleep fits in with the theory. This continual confirmation of the theory through correlational evidence is no proof of its correctness, however, and only a complete understanding of the physiology of sleep will ultimately indicate what it is actually for. The attribution of functions to a process is never easy, boiling down to a matter of understanding and judgement, and scientific ground-rules are rather obscure on this point!

Evolution and Sleep

Field observation and laboratory studies have shown that all vertebrates sleep. The orthodox view of the origins of sleep has been that slow wave sleep (SWS) developed first, and that paradoxical sleep (as REM sleep is called in animals) evolved in warm-blooded animals. Jouvet, for instance, wrote in 1967: '. . . it is at least clear that in the course of evolution slow wave sleep preceded paradoxical sleep. The latter seems to be a more recent acquisition.' Hennevin and Leconte (1971) similarly asserted (author's translation): 'Paradoxical sleep does not exist in fishes, reptiles or amphibians. . . It has been recorded in birds (the chicken, the pigeon), but its proportion is less than 0.3 per cent of orthodox sleep. . . except among predatory birds. . . in fact paradoxical sleep does not appear with all its characteristics except in mammals.'

This has been consistent with the idea that REM sleep is concerned with protein synthesis in the central nervous system (Oswald, 1969) or with memory processes or the elaboration of fixed, instinctive responses (Jouvet, 1963, 1978), in that, obviously, mammals have much better-developed nervous systems than reptiles.

Systematic comparisons of different animals with respect to sleep length, metabolic rate, lifespan, brain weight and other relevant variables made initially by Zepelin and Rechtschaffen (1974) have shown that there is a strong relationship between metabolic rate and total sleep taken over 53 mammalian species. This evidence can be interpreted in terms of sleep being merely a mechanism for reducing energy consumption. Walker and Berger (1980) have argued this, pointing out that animals with high metabolic rates save much-needed energy reserves during sleep. As Oswald (1980) says, it is also consistent with the view that sleep is a period of active recuperation, with high levels of metabolism demanding longer periods of sleep. Oswald has also pointed out that long sleepers among humans have higher body temperatures than have short sleepers (Taub and Berger, 1976), which suggests that longer sleep may be associated with higher metabolic rates even within a species. In this context, the experiments by

Horne, mentioned earlier in the chapter, showing that bodily heating increases stage 4 sleep acquire a new significance, giving support to the Oswald position.

The nature of sleep in animals is obviously of some theoretical importance, and questions of the evolution of sleep and mechanisms of temperature regulation have become crucial issues in the debate about sleep function in man. Some evidence from modern reptiles indicates that their sleep may be more similar to human REM sleep than to human SWS. This would explain the anomaly of the appearance of REM sleep before SWS in the human fetus (when in embryology ontogeny normally follows phylogeny) and the loss of thermoregulation in paradoxical sleep in mammals (Heller and Glotzbach, 1977).

However, there are problems with this analysis in that birds (which show unequivocal SWS) are conventionally viewed as having evolved along with dinosaurs and pterosaurs in parallel to the evolution of mammals from a common primeval reptile. Thus, as Meddis (1983) says, 'the stem reptiles ancestral to birds, mammals, turtles and crocodiles must have been pre-adapted to develop this kind of sleep pattern (SWS) under certain conditions (such as homoeothermy)'. If we follow Desmond (1977) in accepting the persuasive evidence for dinosaurs having been warm-blooded animals, then perhaps this problem could be rationalised by hypothesising a common warm-blooded ancestor to mammals, dinosaurs and birds, which showed SWS, and diverged from the reptilian stem in prehistory. It seems that in this area one man's speculation is as good as another's!

More seriously, actual evidence about the nature of modern reptilian sleep is by no means unambiguous. Most laboratory studies of the EEG of the reptile have shown few signs of slow waves in their periods of quiescence. This has been cited as evidence to suggest that REM sleep is 'reptilian' in origin, and that slow wave sleep is an evolutionarily recent, mammalian development. However, Meglasson and Huggins (1979) found clear evidence of EEG slow waves in 8-month-old crocodiles which were allowed to sunbathe, and they offer the explanation that thermoregulatory behaviour (increasingly recognised as being a major determinant of the temperature of 'cold-blooded' animals) may be necessary for the production of slow wave sleep, and that this may be common to all reptiles, including the ancestral stem reptiles from which birds, mammals, dinosaurs and modern reptiles were evolved. This is a more parsimonious explanation than the ones involving either multiple stem ancestors or preadaptations. That is, all vertebrates share the same sleep mechanisms. So far as the contradictory laboratory evidence goes, as recently as 1971 it was claimed on the basis of EEG recordings that cattle did not sleep at all (Merrick and Scharp, 1971). The experimenters had wired up three steers in individual pens and not one had shown any sign of sleep for 3 days. Any cowman could have told them that cattle hate to sleep alone, and that in a herd there is always one individual awake and standing. Properly conducted experiments subsequently have shown that cattle, like all other mammals, show both REM and slow wave sleep. It seems not unlikely that reptiles are similarly disposed to sleep only when conditions are entirely to their liking, and we must wait for more evidence on reptilian sleep before reaching any firm conclusion.

6

Sleep Disorders

INTRODUCTION

The developments in the study of sleep states outlined early in the last chapter resulted in their being redefined, for all scientific purposes, in terms of EEG. It is, therefore, obviously crucial to a full understanding of the disorders of sleep to know what effect sleep disorders have on EEG-defined sleep patterns. A great deal of work has been carried out over the last 20 years to this end, in recording and assessing the sleep of patients. However, this sort of information is insufficient on its own for the construction of an adequate aetiology of sleep disorders — questions about prevalence, organic origins (sometimes iatrogenic, or caused by medical treatment) and the effects of commonly prescribed drugs are also important.

In the first place, this chapter will be concerned with assessing the severity of the problem of disorders of sleep, and therefore will rely heavily on survey as well as laboratory data. Second, the effects of drugs (especially those taken to deal with sleep problems) must be taken into account, in terms of both frequency of use and their effects on sleep. Only then can one turn to a description of the commonest patterns of sleep disturbance. The classification of sleep disturbance must, therefore, be based on psychophysiological as well as medical criteria, following the recommendations arrived at by the Association of Sleep Disorders Centers (1979).

INSOMNIA AND THE SLEEPING PILL HABIT

Sleep disturbance is extremely common. Bixler *et al.* (1979), in a survey of over 1000 households in Los Angeles, found 38 per cent of their adult respondents complaining of some sleep disorder. They also found that dissatisfaction with sleep increased with age, especially among women. This confirmed the finding of a British survey of a comparable size, conducted in Scotland almost 20 years before (McGhie and Russell, 1962). Bixler *et al.* enquired into the general and mental health correlates of sleep disorder, finding that over 50 per cent of the people complaining of insomnia had other recurring health problems. They were also significantly more likely to complain of tension, loneliness, depression and the need for help with emotional problems, but were not more likely than others to have made any use of mental health facilities. The general picture is thus of sleep disturbance being related to unhappiness, anxiety and poor health. A history of sleep disorder did not make it more likely for an individual to have received treatment for psychiatric illness (although it is, of course, commonplace for people suffering from emotional disorders to also have problems in sleeping).

A second source of information about the prevalence of sleep disorders is the extent of the use of sleeping pills. How many people regularly take a sedative when going to bed? Assessment of the prevalence of use of hypnotics in the general population in Great Britain relies on statistics for the number of prescriptions for various preparations, and on a certain amount of guesswork — first as to the purpose for which the tablets were prescribed, and second as to the proportion actually ingested. At the time of McGhie and Russell's survey in Dundee and Glasgow (1961) the sedatives normally prescribed were barbiturates, and their respondents reported increasing dependence on them with age, especially among women, so that over 25 per cent of women aged 45 and over were in the habit of taking a sedative, while only about 15 per cent of 45-year-old men did so.

More recent estimates of consumption levels (see, e.g., Williams, 1983) reflect a very marked change in prescribing habits over the past 20 years — of 14 million prescriptions for hypnotics in 1960, almost all were for barbiturates, while in 1973 the proportion of non-barbiturate hypnotics prescribed had increased to almost half the total, and by 1978 the barbiturate prescriptions were considerably fewer than half. A continuing survey of the prescribing habits of all 859 doctors who entered general practice in the year 1969/1970 clearly shows that by 1976 barbiturates were prescribed essentially only to patients who had become dependent on them, by these recently qualified GPs, and practically all new prescriptions for hypnotics were of the non-barbiturate variety (Birmingham Research Unit, 1978).

Information about prescribing levels tells us when certain drugs cease to be prescribed (like the barbiturates) but does not necessarily indicate which other drugs took their place. This problem is particularly acute with the hypnotics, since so many preparations can be prescribed to patients who complain of sleeplessness. Rare evidence of the medical response to patients presenting themselves with 'insomnia' is given by a survey of five GPs at the Aldermoor Health Centre, attached to the Southampton University Medical School (Freeman, 1978). Of the 250 patients dealt with, only 4 were prescribed barbiturates, and the most popular drugs were nitrazepam (Mogadon), diazepam (Valium) and other benzodiazepines. However, almost half of the prescriptions for the under-14s were for antihistamines, and almost a third of those for the

over-65s were for chlormethiazole, a powerful barbiturate-like sedative. (It is
known that some milder drugs, such as nitrazepam, can cause confusion and
dementia in the elderly, so these rather potent sedatives represent the lesser of
two evils for these patients.) Chloral derivatives and antidepressants were also
given quite often, the former mainly to the under-14s, the latter to patients in
middle age or older.

Therefore, no single group of preparations can be classed as 'hypnotic', as
doctors obviously attempt to match prescriptions to patients' specific needs, and
make use of a wide variety of drugs. This flexibility in usage means that data for
the number and types of prescription must be interpreted with some caution.
Over the years the benzodiazepines have become the most widely used psychotropic drugs, with the total number of prescriptions dispensed in Great Britain
levelling off at about 30 million by the mid-1970s. About 13 million of these
were accounted for by these marketed as hypnotics. However, an unknown
number of the remaining 17 million 'anxiolytics' will have been prescribed as
hypnotics — in the Freeman study diazepam was freely prescribed as a hypnotic
— and, of course, the use that patients make of these drugs is also obscure. Some
indication of trends in prescribing over the 10 year period up to 1983 is given by
the graph in Figure 6.1. A general increase in the dispensation of anxiolytic

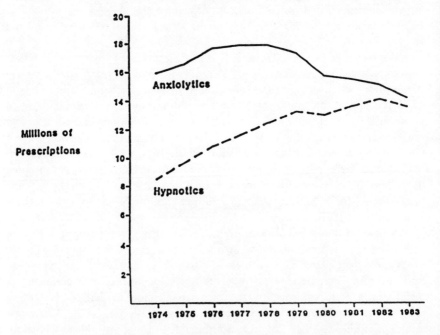

Figure 6.1 Prescribing levels for benzodiazepines, 1974–1983. Based on a sample of 1 in
200 prescriptions in England and Wales and 1 in 100 in Scotland — dispensed in contracting
chemists' establishments (including drug stores) and by appliance contractors. Data supplied
by DHSS Statistical and Research Division

benzodiazepines (marketed as anti-anxiety drugs, normally intended to be taken during the day) from the 1960s peaked in 1977. Over the following 6 years their prescription showed a pronounced drop, while the number of prescriptions for hypnotics continued to rise. This may reflect an increasing tendency to prescribe specifically 'hypnotic' benzodiazepine drugs for sleep problems, rather than diazepam (e.g. Valium) or chlordiazepoxide (e.g. Librium).

Recent changes in regulations in the UK, designed to reduce the costs to the National Health Service of branded drugs by disallowing named preparations, will undoubtedly affect prescribing patterns in the future. For instance, the two most widely prescribed hypnotic benzodiazepines (nitrazepam and flurazepam) will only be permitted in tablet form, not capsules, presumably because capsules are only available in branded form — and the brand names associated with these two preparations, Mogadon and Dalmane, are specifically banned from NHS prescriptions, along with most other brand names. More importantly, while well-established products will be available in generic form, new drugs will not, so a probable result of these regulations will be the slowing of the introduction of new drugs in the UK.

Official statistics on prescribing levels cannot provide more than a very rough guide to the prevalence of people taking hypnotic drugs — that is, drugs taken to improve sleep quality — and the only reliable way of finding out how many people do so is to systematically ask them. A survey of psychotropic drug consumption in the general population carried out in 1977 (Murray *et al.*, 1981) found that only 11 per cent of adults had taken 'sedatives' in a 2 week period, the same as that found 8 years previously by Dunnell and Cartwright (1972), despite a large increase over the same period in the number of prescriptions. Cartwright (1980) suggests that there has been a decline in the proportion of patients taking the drugs prescribed to them, and also the development of a degree of scepticism towards medical authority between 1969 and 1977, so that patients became more likely to take drugs as they felt the need for them rather than as the doctor ordered.

However, despite the lower than expected levels of consumption, the survey of Murray *et al.* confirmed previous British and American evidence (McGhie and Russell, 1962; Bixler *et al.*, 1979) that women are very much more likely to take hypnotics than men, and that this difference increases with age. This finding paradoxically contradicts laboratory evidence about the quality of sleep achieved, in general, by elderly men and women in the laboratory. There, men have almost twice as many wakenings and disturbances during the night as do women, and, objectively, it would seem likely that a greater proportion of men would become dissatisfied with their sleep to the extent of demanding hypnotics. Are women generally more neurotic than men as they get older, or is this specifically a sleep problem? The evidence of Murray *et al.* shows that the proportion of women taking anxiolytic drugs actually decreased with age, which demonstrates a lack of association between sleep disorder and general anxiety level, and contradicts an interpretation that the increase in sleep disorders with age among women is symptomatic of a higher general level of neuroticism as women get older. No simple explanation can be offered for this sex difference.

THE SLEEP OF INSOMNIACS

Psychophysiological studies of the sleep of insomniacs — that is, of people who complain of sleeping badly — have consistently shown that self-report of sleep quality does not predict quantity or quality of sleep, as assessed in the laboratory, at all reliably. Most people overestimate the time it takes to get to sleep (Lewis, 1969). Insomniacs tend to have longer latencies to sleep onset, and do achieve less overall sleep than normal controls (Monroe, 1967; Karacan *et al.*, 1971). However, their complaints of lack of sleep or of failure to get to sleep may often seem out of proportion to the psychophysiological evidence, and some insomniacs will even report wakefulness when roused from stage 4 sleep (Rechtschaffen and Monroe, 1969).

Recent work (Hauri and Olmstead, 1983) has shown that the best estimate of an insomniac's definition of sleep onset is the beginning of the first 15 min of uninterrupted stage 2 sleep, rather than stage 2 sleep onset *per se*, which they confirmed as being the best estimate of subjective sleep onset in normals. Not only, therefore, do insomniacs achieve less or worse sleep than normals, but also perception of it exacerbates the problem. Some people demanding sedatives may not be deprived of sleep at all, but only of the experience of unconsciousness. Many 'normals' have less sleep than most 'insomniacs', without complaint. Gaillard (1975) expressed this fourfold typology very neatly in a diagram (see Figure 6.2).

Short Sleepers

A group of people distinct from insomniacs are those who never seem to need very much sleep, and generally do not complain to the medical profession about their sleep, although they sleep 5 h or less. Assessment of the severity of any sleep disorder must be based on an idea of how much sleep, and what sort of sleep, people actually need. Short sleepers are highly interesting in this respect. Jones and Oswald (1968) studied the sleep of two Australian men who claimed normally to sleep for less than 2 h, and in the laboratory it was confirmed that they did, in fact, sleep very little. More important, the patterning of their sleep was unusual, in that stages 3, 4 and REM accounted for over 70 per cent of total sleep — a much greater proportion than in normals. Hartmann *et al.* (1971) recruited subjects by newspaper advertisement who claimed to sleep more than 9 or less than 6 h, and found that although these groups differed greatly in the total amount of sleep they achieved in the laboratory, both groups took the same amount of stage 4 sleep, and similar percentages of REM sleep. These findings are consistent with the view that, while much light sleep (stages 1 and 2) is, so to speak, optional, it is important to achieve a certain minimal amount of REM sleep and deep slow wave sleep (stages 3 and 4).

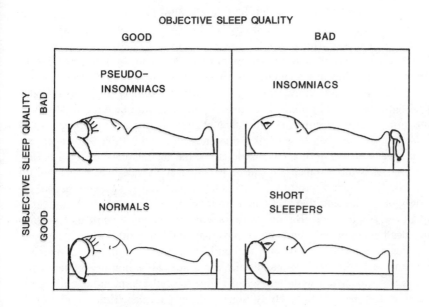

Figure 6.2 Types of sleepers. Satisfaction with sleep need not correlate well with objectively determined sleep quality

DISORDERS OF INITIATING SLEEP

Almost half of the people in Bixler's survey who reported insomnia had difficulty in falling asleep. Worry and anxiety are commonly given as reasons for not falling asleep. However, contrary to this usual view that it is anxiety which causes difficulties in falling asleep, normal levels of anxiety and stress do not seem to have any simple effect on sleep latency in the laboratory. Haynes *et al.* (1981) stressed insomniacs and non-insomniacs with mental arithmetic problems after lights-out in the laboratory, and found no consistent effect on time taken to get to sleep afterwards — the insomniacs taking slightly shorter than before and the non-insomniacs taking considerably longer. Freedman and Sattler (1982) specifically studied the mental content of sleep onset insomniacs, to compare it with that of non-insomniacs. Many of their patients had complained of being 'unable to fall asleep because [they] could not turn off [their] mind'. Psychophysiological measures of autonomic arousal taken before lights-out, and mental content reports of the period before sleep onset, did not provide convincing evidence that worry or anxiety was *causing* the real delay in sleep onset shown by their insomniacs (44 min versus 13 min in the controls). They conclude that 'excessive rumination may be an epiphenomenon of sleeplessness' rather than its cause.

Similarly, while Rosa *et al*. (1983), in a study of subjects selected as being highly anxious, found them to sleep slightly less, more lightly and with fewer wakenings than a control group, their sleep latency was unaffected. The relationship between anxiety and this sleep disorder is obviously not simple. Priest (1978) reports that in his clinical experience strong emotions of resentment or anger will more commonly prevent sleep than will anxiety. He suggest that in persistent cases of sleep onset insomnia, attention should be directed at sources of conflict causing resentment rather than at any resulting sleep problems.

Very high levels of anxiety or worry must be incompatible with sleep, and sleep always suffers during psychiatric crises, but the relationship between sleep and arousal is not simple, and can be paradoxical. Oswald (1959) pointed out how bodily restraints and rhythmic stimulation can induce 'animal hypnosis' in a variety of species, and that this state of immobility was known to be accompanied by EEG signs of sleep. His own experiments on human volunteers confirmed that sleep could be induced in conditions that could only otherwise be described as highly arousing. All this is consistent with the Pavlovian notion that impossible tasks or very disagreeable conditions can result in 'inhibitory experimental neuroses' — including withdrawal and sleep. A similar explanation, applied to infantile sleep behaviour by Harry Stack Sullivan (Sullivan, 1953), is that of the 'dynamism of somnolent detachment'.

A recent interpretation of the aetiology of sleep onset insomnia has been Weitzman's suggestion that it is caused by a disturbance of biological rhythm. This syndrome, of regularly not going to bed until the early hours of the morning, and then being unwilling to get up until lunch-time, is quite common among students. These individuals are clearly getting plenty of sleep, but at the wrong time of day. The draconian cure proposed for such people with a chronic inability to fall asleep at a particular clock time ('chronotherapy') is to reset their circadian rhythms with a progressive phase delay of bed-time by 3 h each week until the desired bed-time is arrived at (Weitzman, 1981). However, it is unclear how many patients have been sufficiently persistent (and have had sufficiently flexible life-styles) to complete the course of treatment.

To sum up, difficulty in getting to sleep can sometimes be attributed to excessive levels of anxiety (in particular, apprehension about forthcoming and potentially stressful events), but is commonly caused either by feelings of resentment accompanied by rumination or by the lack of any pressure for sleep.

DISORDERS OF MAINTAINING SLEEP

Almost three-quarters of the insomniacs studied by Bixler *et al*. reported difficulty in staying asleep, and just under half reported early wakening. These two symptoms both increased in frequency with age, especially the early wakenings. Arousals to light stage 1 sleep or wakefulness typically occur at the end of REM sleep periods in normals (Langford *et al.*, 1972) but are not usually remembered, because they are brief. Wakenings have to be longer than 2 min or so to be clearly recalled next day.

Lightened sleep and relatively early wakenings are normal features of old age, and are not normally associated with day-time sleepiness. Persistent maintenance insomnia in middle age or earlier is commonly associated with affective illness, drug abuse, alcoholism and respiratory illnesses. Both monopolar and bipolar affective disorders are associated with shortened REM latency (time between sleep onset and the first REM sleep period) and reduced stages 3 and 4. Monopolar depression is also associated with reduced sleep, repeated wakenings and early arousal (Kupfer, 1976; Gillin *et al.*, 1979). The classic relationships between endogenous depression and early wakening, and between exogenous depression and failure to initiate sleep, have never been confirmed, despite the fact that these considerations have presumably been taken into account whenever these sorts of diagnoses have been made (Costello and Selby, 1965; Mendels and Hawkins, 1967).

A minority of patients complaining of insomnia actually suffer from 'alpha-delta' sleep, first identified by Hauri and Hawkins (1973), in which the EEG patterns of wakefulness (the 10 Hz alpha rhythm) persist during slow wave sleep and the 12–15 Hz spindling of stage 2 is superimposed on the low-voltage mixed-frequency EEG of stage REM sleep. These patients report not having slept at all and feel that they derive little benefit from sleep, although they regularly sleep uninterruptedly for 6 h or more. This syndrome is characteristic of patients suffering from fibrositis, as described in Chapter 5.

The routine use of a measure of respiration in the night-time assessment of the sleep of patients complaining of maintenance insomnia led Guilleminault *et al.* (1973) to discover that the causation of insomnia in a few of them was entirely respiratory. Not only that, but this fact was unknown to them or their doctors, and, typically, they had a lengthy history of taking a variety of hypnotics which only exacerbated their problems. These people suffer from sleep apnoea, in which respiration ceases during sleep until the build-up of carbon dioxide in blood causes them to wake up gasping for air. Peripheral airway obstruction can be implicated as the primary cause in a minority of patients, and in these surgery can provide a total cure of the problem. No cure can be suggested at present for central sleep apnoea, which seems to be an innate central nervous system malfunction, but hypnotics are obviously no help, and can gradually be withdrawn.

Allen *et al.* (1971) report that alcoholics drying out and suffering from delirium tremens will have fitful sleep for 6–8 days with 50–100 per cent REM sleep accompanied by hallucinatory dreams. Disturbances of sleep will continue for up to 6 months after the first 'good night's sleep', however, with delayed sleep onset and multiple wakenings through the night. Essentially similar symptoms result from withdrawal from the barbiturates (Oswald and Priest, 1965). Kales *et al.* (1969) have argued that tolerance to CNS depressants (such as alcohol, barbiturates and the opiates) produces a syndrome of its own — Drug Dependency Insomnia — and any beneficial sleep-inducing properties of, for instance, barbiturate hypnotics are lost after a few weeks' use.

Drugs taken initially to deal with transient sleep problems (such as sleep onset insomnia caused by some life crisis) can thus become the mainstay of a drug-dependent pattern of sleep — inducing a classic teratogenic illness, where a course of medical treatment causes an illness in its own right.

Lastly, maintenance insomnia may be caused by periodic jerking movements in Ekbom's 'restless legs syndrome'. These are persistent and exaggerated forms of the twitches (myoclonal jerks) that most people occasionally experience on going to sleep, often associated with sensations of falling. In this condition they occur every 20–30 s during slow wave sleep, disrupting sleep onset, and causing disturbance throughout the night. There is no known cure for this condition, and, as with sleep apnoea, heavy sedation is not beneficial.

DISORDERS OF AROUSAL

A group of disorders — somnambulism, enuresis and night terrors — have been classified together by Broughton (1968) as being disorders of autonomic arousal associated with slow wave sleep.

Somnambulism is fairly common. Anders and Weinstein (1972) report that 15 per cent of all children have had at least one episode, and between 1 and 6 per cent suffer from frequent attacks. Typically, the subject sits up in bed, or gets up, in stage 3 or 4 sleep, following some particularly large paroxysmal slow waves in EEG (Kales *et al.*, 1966). Usually the episode lasts less than 15 min, and after some apparently non-purposive, often repetitive activity the subject either goes back to sleep — often in his or her own bed — or wakes up. There is anecdotal evidence that this disorder runs in families. For instance, a student who consulted the author about problems caused by sleepwalking in her hall of residence revealed that the whole of her family had once woken up in the early hours of the morning seated around the kitchen table, where they had all happened to congregate in their sleep. Anders and Weinstein suggest that enuresis and night terrors as well as somnambulism may be genetically associated.

Enuresis is, of course, invariable in babies. 'Primary' enuresis is defined as the persistence of bed-wetting into childhood and 'secondary' enuresis as its reappearance after a period of successful bladder continence. Broughton (1968) estimates that 10–15 per cent of 'nervous' children and 30 per cent of institutionalised children wet their beds, and cites evidence indicating that 1 per cent of US naval recruits are enuretic (despite screening for this among other disorders), as are 24 per cent of naval recruits discharged on psychiatric grounds. Anders and Weinstein (1972) confirm, as these figures would suggest, that enuresis is associated with emotional stress, and often reappears as late as adolescence. Enuresis typically occurs after a period of deep slow wave sleep

(Broughton, 1968). Recordings of pressure in the bladder showed that bed-wetting is preceded by an increasingly strong series of bladder contractions (which could also be stimulated by clicks, hand-claps or other noises), quite unlike the pattern of bladder pressures recorded in normal controls. These excessive contractions did not always result in bed-wetting, but invariably preceded those episodes that were recorded, which also always occurred during slow wave sleep arousals.

Nightmares should be distinguished from night terrors, in that they consist of a frightening dream concerning some anxiety-laden topic and normally occur during REM sleep. Waking up from an anxiety nightmare of this sort can be just as frightening as waking up from a night terror, with the difference that re-assurance is possible, as the fear is caused by the subject matter and plot of the dream. With night terrors it seems that the fear comes first, with no 'supporting' dream scenario. Typically, a child wakes its parents with an ear-splitting scream, and remains inconsolably terrified for ten or fifteen minutes before falling back again into a deep sleep. Next morning only the parents can remember the incident. Adults can also suffer from night terrors, although less commonly and less spectacularly.

Another, related, disorder of arousal is sleep paralysis, in which the flaccid paralysis of REM sleep intrudes into wakefulness. Attacks last up to 10 min, and can occur at sleep onset or during the night's sleep at the end of an REM sleep period. Sleep paralysis can in itself be very frightening — especially if accom-panied by hallucinations or preceded by a nightmare. The idea of pressure on the chest, or immobility, in the notions of 'incubus' and 'cauchmar' signifying being lain upon, and pressing down upon, must surely refer to sleep paralysis rather than the other two varieties of nightmare. It is, of course, very common indeed in patients suffering from narcolepsy (being one of the four defining symptoms associated in this syndrome) but is also relatively common in normal adolescence. Goode (1962) found that 5 per cent of a sample of medical and nursing students reported sleep paralysis as having occurred at least once in the past year. People who regularly suffer from attacks may gain some 'lucidity', so that they recognise what is happening to them and wait for the resumption of control over their bodies in relative tranquillity (Hishikawa, 1976).

THE HYPERSOMNIAS

Excessive day-time sleepiness may be the result of a lack of adequate night-time sleep, caused by, for example, pain, jet-lag or the effects of stimulant drugs at night. Sleep apnoea is incompatible with normal sleep patterns, and most patients studied by Guilleminault *et al.* (1973) suffering from sleep apnoea also com-plained of sleepiness during the day.

Permanent sleepiness may be a symptom of narcolepsy. This is a condition characterised by a tetrad of symptoms — sleep attacks and day-time somnolence, cataplexy, hypnagogic hallucinations and sleep paralysis. The study of the EEG of narcoleptic patients has been crucial in furthering understanding of this disorder. Night-time sleep is essentially normal, with the important difference that wakefulness is typically immediately followed by REM sleep rather than a steady progression through the slow wave sleep stages (Rechtschaffen *et al.*, 1963). The tendency to do this is more marked in patients who also complain of cataplexy, and is common in day-time sleep attacks and night-time sleep onset.

Cataplexy is an extreme form of the helplessness that can be induced in anybody laughing hilariously or being 'tickled to death'. Any extreme of emotion causes narcoleptics to fall down, with flaccid paralysis of all muscles except the respiratory and oculomotor ones, just as in REM sleep. Hypnagogic hallucinations, the visual and auditory images that many people experience with the onset of sleep, are always reported by narcoleptics. Sleep paralysis, as noted above, is common in adolescence, but persists throughout life in patients suffering from narcolepsy, and is a wakening in which the flaccid paralysis of REM sleep is maintained.

THE EFFECTS OF HYPNOTIC DRUGS

The dramatic change in prescribing habits in hypnotics in the late 1960s was not only a response to the epidemic of deaths through overdosing and the availability of relatively non-toxic alternatives, but also because of advances in understanding of the effects of barbiturates on sleep and of their addictiveness, gained through EEG studies. Oswald and Priest (1965) showed that barbiturates reduce the amount of REM sleep when first taken, like many other drugs. As tolerance developed over a few days, the level of REM sleep returned to normal, but on withdrawal the habitual user experienced vivid dreams and nightmares, with frequent night-time wakenings caused by a massive REM sleep rebound, with double the usual amount of REM sleep, lasting for five or six weeks. These symptoms may often have led patients to return to their doctors to ask for repeat prescriptions of the sedatives, ensuring a drug-dependent way of life in an otherwise healthy person.

There have been a good number of EEG studies of the effects of various hypnotics on sleep, but not all of them have been as extended as they, perhaps, ought to have been, or have used appropriate subjects. Prescriptions for hypnotics are usually for a fortnight or a month, and may be repeated many times. The time course of drug use and recovery is normally of the order of weeks rather than days. However, most empirical studies of the psychophysiological effects of these drugs only take recordings for a week or so – typically, two nights' baseline recordings, three nights on medication and three nights' recovery. This may be sufficient to give an indication of the pharmacological action of the preparation, but cannot be taken very seriously as ecologically valid data about the effects of the drug in the real world. An honourable exception to the snapshot approach is the work of Ernest Hartmann, who, in a series of experiments published in 1976, studied the effects of a variety of drugs on sleep, taking periods of drug use of 3 weeks rather than 3 days and following up for up to 6 weeks after withdrawal. Another fault of many laboratory studies of the effects of hypnotics on sleep is that they usually involve healthy volunteers in their early twenties – typically, university students. The majority of patients receiving medication for sleep problems are over 40, and many are quite elderly. It is, admittedly, difficult to recruit older people to sleep laboratory experiments – perhaps the development of home recording systems will facilitate this sort of research in the future.

Chlordiazepoxide (a minor tranquilliser, or benzodiazepine, marketed in the UK as Librium) increases the time spent asleep without reducing REM sleep (Hartmann, 1968). It has also been found to reduce the amount of deep slow wave sleep (stage 4), and over long periods there is evidence that REM sleep may be reduced (Hartmann, 1976). However, after a month of drugged sleep in that study, there was no strong evidence of REM rebound in a recovery month.

Chloral hydrate, like the barbiturates, suppresses REM sleep initially, and causes a massive rebound on withdrawal (Hartmann, 1976). However, it is rapidly metabolised, unlike either the benzodiazepines or barbiturates, whose half-lives in the body are between 14 and 30 h.

Amitryptyline, an antidepressant of the tricyclic variety frequently prescribed to patients presenting with sleep problems, has been shown to slightly increase total sleep time, to reduce REM sleep time with no adaptation over a 30 day period, and to cause a relatively short-lived REM sleep rebound on withdrawal (Hartmann, 1976). Monoamine oxidase inhibitors (antidepressants acting directly on brain metabolism) actually abolish REM sleep as they take effect on the patient's mood, and it has even been proposed (Dunleavy and Oswald, 1973; Vogel *et al.*, 1975) that it is the deprivation of REM sleep that brings the thera- peutic effect. The tricyclics also depress REM sleep, but adaptation occurs over a few nights, and REM returns to normal levels.

Most hypnotics have a long half-life in blood, so that their effects are not confined to the night, if taken in the evening. Walters and Lader (1970) have shown that both a benzodiazepine and a barbiturate can depress performance on simple psychomotor tasks on the day following administration – not surprisingly, perhaps, in the case of the barbiturate, but somewhat unexpectedly in the case of the benzodiazepine, which is normally credited with tranquillising without sedating. Benzodiazepines with short half-lives (3–5 h) have been developed recently (such as temazepam) but have not received overwhelmingly enthusiastic medical approval, perhaps because they are (by definition) ineffective in main- taining their hypnotic effect over a whole night, while the more commonly prescribed drugs, such as nitrazepam, build up over a period of days. None of these drugs is ideal, but the benzodiazepines are perhaps the least harmful, and are the hypnotics most likely to be prescribed by doctors in the UK.

SLEEP DISORDERS CLINICS

It has already been pointed out that people are not very accurate in their recollections of wakenings during the night, or the delay to sleep onset, or of whether they were asleep (according to EEG criteria) or awake. Even the most conscientious physician, therefore, is at a disadvantage when attempting to make a diagnosis of primary insomnia on the basis of a patient's self-report.

In the USA a number of sleep disorders clinics have been founded, offering routine polysomnographic assessment, and their collective experience has been summarised in a systematic classification of sleep disorders (Association of Sleep Disorders Centers, 1979).

Ancoli-Israel *et al.* (1981) report on the effects of referral to such a clinic of 170 consecutive patients. One hundred and seventeen of them were deemed to require polysomnographic assessment. Fifty-one of these were found to have sleep apnoea, which was obstructive in origin in 37. Patients with apnoea were significantly older than those without (52 compared with 42 years), and a good number of them were obese. Nine were treated with tracheostomy, which was successful for eight of them. Eight patients were admitted and treated with a strict reducing diet, and three of the four who did achieve normal weights had fewer apnoeic attacks. The seriousness of this condition is demonstrated by the fact that two of these patients died in their sleep, one of them at the age of 47 with no other medically recognised disease. Twelve patients assessed in the clinic suffered from uncomplicated nocturnal myoclonus (Ekbom's syndrome). Twenty-nine other patients were given specific diagnoses of sleep disorders related to depression, drug abuse, organic brain disease or hypochondriasis.

In summing up the benefits of the clinic, Ancoli-Israel *et al.* stress the importance of discouraging unnecessary referrals and limiting polysomnography to those patients 'for whom a clinical indication is strong', and ascribe their success in achieving specific diagnoses in 90 per cent of the patients recorded to this selectivity. Several of the patients suffering from sleep apnoeas or narcolepsy were able to resume work, with treatment appropriate to their conditions. None of the patients given treatment actually died in the course of the study, while five of the untreated patients died. It is clear that a few patients can benefit enormously from this sort of assessment, and after a lifetime of taking inappropriate but highly potent drugs can at last be given some real relief from their symptoms.

Rather mysteriously, the incidence of sleep apnoea in the UK is extremely low (Shapiro *et al.*, 1981). Since it is only in the apnoeic syndrome that polysomnographic evidence is crucial in making a diagnosis, this could be taken as an argument for not pursuing this sort of assessment, which is both costly and laborious. However, in view of the prevalence of the suffering caused by sleep disorders in general, and the widespread use of hypnotics, it could be argued that some relatively inexpensive system of recording EEG, EOG, EMG and respiration at home would improve both the accuracy of diagnosis and the suitability of prescribing in those patients who seem to be chronically in need of sedation. This could be a service provided by psychologists attached to group practices or health services. A postal survey of all the general practitioners in the Hull area in 1979 showed that there was firm support for a proposed service like this among a sizeable majority of the respondents, and that a referral rate of three or four patients per year could be expected from each of these doctors — more than enough demand to employ a psychologist and two or three nurses.

Enough is now known about the aetiology of sleep disorders to show that the palliatives offered in the past have been ineffective, and in some cases positively harmful. While there have certainly been great pharmacological improvements, in that modern sedatives are rarely lethal in overdose and are non-addictive in themselves, relatively little has been done to develop polysomnography and provide ordinary clinicians with understandable information about the sleep of their patients.

This chapter has been an account of the undoubted success of EEG in uncovering the true nature of the disorders of sleep. It is unfortunate that it cannot report on any widespread application of these techniques in the assessment of insomniacs, or even the systematic assessment of hypnotic drugs on appropriate groups of people over appropriate lengths of time.

References

Adam, K. (1980). Sleep as a restorative process and a theory to explain why. *Prog. Brain Res.*, **53**, 289

Adrian, E. D. and Matthews, B. H. C. (1934). The Berger rhythm: potential changes from the occipital lobes of man. *Brain*, **57**, 355

Adrian, E. D. and Yamigawa, K. (1935). The origin of the Berger rhythm. *Brain*, **58**, 323

Agnew, H., Webb, W. and Williams, R. (1964). The effect of stage four sleep deprivation. *EEG Jl*, **17**. 68

Allen, R. P. *et al.* (1971). EEG sleep recovery following prolonged alcohol intoxication in alcoholics. *J. Nerv. Ment. Dis.*, **152**, 424

Allison, T., Wood, C. C. and Goff, W. R. (1983). Brain-stem auditory, pattern-reversal visual, and short-latency somatosensory EPs – Latencies in relation to age, sex and size. *EEG Jl.*, **55**, 619

Anand, B., Chhina, G. and Singh, B. (1961). Some aspects of electroencephalographic studies in Yogis. *EEG Jl.*, **13**, 452

Ancoli-Israel, S. *et al.* (1981). Benefits of a sleep disorders clinic in a veterans administration medical center. *West. J. Med.*, **135**, 14

Anders, T. F. and Weinstein, P. (1972). Sleep and disorders in infants and children – a review. *Pediatrics*, **50**, 312

Andersen, P. and Andersson, S. A. (1968). *Physiological Basis of the Alpha Rhythm.* Appleton Century Crofts, New York

Aserinsky, E. and Kleitman, N. (1953). Regularly occurring periods of eye motility, and concomitant phenomena, during sleep. *Science, N.Y.*, **118**, 273

Association of Sleep Disorders Centers (1979). Diagnostic classification of sleep and arousal disorders. *Sleep*, **2**, 1

Baekeland, F. and Laski, R. (1966). Exercise and sleep patterns in college athletes. *Percept. Motor Skills*, **23**, 1203

Banquet, J. P. (1973). Spectral analysis of the EEG in meditation. *EEG Jl.*, **35**, 143

Barber, T. X. (1969). *Hypnosis: A Scientific Approach.* Van Nostrand, New York

Barker, W. and Burgwin, S. (1949). Brain wave patterns during hypnosis, hypnotic sleep and normal sleep. *Arch. Neurol. Psychiat.*, **62**, 412

Barwood, T. *et al.* (1978). Auditory evoked potentials and transcendental meditation. *EEG Jl*, **45**, 671

Beatty, J. (1972). Similar effects of feedback signals and instructional information on EEG activity. *Physiol. Behav.*, **9**, 151

Beaumont, J. G. (Ed.) (1981). *Divided Visual Field Studies of Cerebral Organisation.* Academic Press, London

Beaumont, J. G. (1983). The EEG and task performance: a tutorial review. In Gaillard, A. W. K. and Ritter, W. (Eds.), *Tutorials in Event Related Potential Research.* North-Holland, Amsterdam

Beck, A. (1890). Die Bestimmung der Localization der Gehirn- und Ruckenmarkfunctionen vermittelst der electrischen Erscheinungen. *Zbl. Physiol.*, **4**, 473

Bell, G. A. and Van Ireland, G. H. C. R. M. (1976). Interhemispheric asymmetry of alpha waves. *Rep. Psychol. Labs, La Trobe Univ.*, **1**, 35

Benson, H. (1976). *The Relaxation Response*. Collins, London

Berger, H. (1929). Uber das Ellektrenkephalogramm des Menschen. *Arch. Psychiat. NervKrankh.*, **87**, 527

Berger, R. J. and Oswald, I. (1962). Effects of sleep deprivation on behaviour, subsequent sleep, and dreaming. *J. Ment. Sci.*, **108**, 457

Bernhard, C. G. and Skoglund, C. R. (1943). On the blocking of the cortical alpha rhythm in children. *Acta Psychiat. Neurol.*, **18**, 159

Binnie, C. D., Rowan, A. J. and Gutter, T. H. (1982). *A Manual of Electro-encephalographic Technology*. Cambridge University Press, Cambridge

Birmingham Research Unit of the Royal College of General Practitioners (1978). Practice activity analysis, 4. Psychotropic drugs. *J. Roy. Coll. Gen. Pract.*, **28**, 122

Bixler, E. O. *et al.* (1979). Prevalence of sleep disorders in the Los Angeles metropolitan area. *Am. J. Psychiat.*, **136**, 1257

Blinkhorn, S. F. and Hendrickson, D. E. (1982). Averaged evoked responses and psychometric intelligence. *Nature, Lond.*, **295**, 596

Boddy, J. (1971). The relationship of reaction to brain wave periods: a re-evaluation of the evidence. *EEG Jl*, **30**, 229

Bradley, C. and Meddis, R. (1974). Arousal threshold in dreaming sleep. *Physiol. Psychol.*, **2**, 109

Brazier, M. A. B. (1961). *A History of the Electrical Activity of the Brain*. Macmillan, New York

Bremer, F. (1937). L'activité cerebrale au cours du sommeil et de la narcose contribution à l'étude du mecanisme du sommeil. *Bull. Acad. Roy. Med. Belg.*, **2**, 68

Brezinova, V. and Oswald, I. (1972). Sleep after a bedtime beverage. *Br. Med. J.*, **2**, 431

Broadbent, D. E. (1971). *Decision and Stress*. Academic Press, New York

Brooker, B. H. and Donald, M. W. (1980). Contribution of the speech musculature to apparent human EEG asymmetries prior to vocalization. *Brain Lang.*, **9**, 226

Broughton, R. J. (1968). Sleep disorders: disorders of arousal? *Science, N.Y.*, **159**, 1070

Broughton, R. J., Regis, H. and Gastaut, H. (1964). Modification of somaesthetic evoked potentials during bursts of mu rhythm and fist clenching. *EEG Jl*, **18**, 720 [abstract]

Brown, B. (1970). Recognition of aspects of consciousness through association with EEG alpha rhythm. *Psychophysiology*, **6**, 442

Brown, I. D. (1961). Measuring the spare 'mental capacity' of cardrivers by a subsidiary task. *Ergonomics*, **4**, 35

Brunia, C. H. M. and Vingerhoets, A. J. J. M. (1981). Opposite hemisphere differences in movement–related potentials preceding foot and finger movements. *Biol. Psychol.*, **13**, 261

Bunnell, D. E., Bevier, W. and Horvath, S. M. (1983). Effects of exhaustive exercise on the sleep of men and women. *Psychophysiology*, **20**, 50

Butler, C. H. M. and Glass, A. (1976). EEG correlates of cerebral dominance. In Riesen, A. H. and Thompson, R. F. (Eds.), *Advances in Psychobiology*, Vol. 3, pp. 219–272. Wiley, New York

Callaway, E. (1962). Factors influencing the relationship between alpha activity and visual reaction time. *EEG Jl*, **14**, 674

Carskadon, M. A. and Dement, W. C. (1975). Sleep studies on a 90-minute day. *EEG Jl*, **39**, 145

Cartwright, A. (1980). Prescribing and the patient–doctor relationship. In Hasler, J. and Pendleton, D. (Eds.), *Essays on Doctor–Patient Communication*. Academic Press, London

Caton, R. (1875). The electric currents of the brain. *Br. Med. J.*, **2**, 278

Cavonius, C. R. and Estevez–Uscaryn, D. (1974). Local suppression of alpha activity by pattern in half the visual field. *Nature, Lond.*, **251**, 412

Chatrian, G. E. (1976). The mu rhythm. In Remond, A. (Ed.), *Handbook of Electro-encephalography and Clinical Neurophysiology*, Vol. 6. North-Holland, Amsterdam

Chatrian, G. E., Petersen, M. C. and Lazarte, J. A. (1959). The blocking of the rolandic wicket rhythm and some central changes related to movement. *EEG Jl*, **11**, 497

Chertok, L. and Kramarz, P. (1959). Hypnosis, sleep and electroencephalography. *J. Nerv. Ment. Dis.*, **128**, 227

Clarke, L. G. and Harding, F. A. (1969). Comparisons of mono and dizygotic twins with respect to some features of the electro-encephalogram. *Proc. Electrophys. Technol. Ass.*, **16**, 94

Costello, C. G. and Selby, M. M. (1965). The relationship between sleep patterns and reactive and endogenous depression. *Br. J. Psychiat.*, **111**, 497

Craik, F. I. M. and Lockhardt, R. S. (1972). Levels of processing: A framework for memory research. *J. Verb. Learn. Verb. Behav.*, **11**, 671

Crick, F. and Mitchison, G. (1983). The function of dreaming. *Nature, Lond.*, **304**, 111

Crisp, A. H. and Stonehill, E. (1977). *Sleep, Nutrition and Mood*. Wiley, London

Dement, W. C. (1960). The effect of dream deprivation. *Science, N. Y.*, **131**, 1705

Dement, W. C. (1974). *Some Must Watch While Some Must Sleep*. Freeman, San Francisco

Dement, W. C. and Wolpert, E. A. (1958). The relation of eye movements, body motility, and external stimuli to dream content. *J. Exp. Psychol.*, **55**, 543

Desmedt, J. E. and Robertson, D. (1977). Differential enhancement of early and late components of the cerebral somato-sensory potentials during cognitive tasks. *J. Physiol.*, **271**, 761

Desmond, A. J. (1977). *The Hot-Blooded Dinosaurs*. Futura, London

Donchin, E. (1981). Surprise!. . . . .Surprise! Presidential address, Society for Psychophysiological Research. *Psychophysiology*, **18**, 493

Donchin, E., Kutas, M. and McCarthy, G. (1977). Electrocortical indices of hemispheric utilization. In Harnad, S. *et al.* (Eds.), *Lateralization in the Nervous System*, pp. 339–384. Academic Press, New York

Du Bois-Reymond, E. (1848). *Untersuchungen uber thierische Elektricitat*. Reimer, Berlin

Duffy, E. (1934). Emotion: An example of the need for reorientation in psychology. *Psychol. Rev.*, **41**, 184

Dunleavy, D. L. F. and Oswald, I. (1973). Phenelzine, mood response and sleep. *Arch. Gen. Psychiat.*, **28**, 353

Dunnell, K. and Cartwright, A. (1972). *Medicine Takers, Prescribers and Hoarders*. Routledge and Kegan Paul, London

Dustman, R. E. and Beck, E. C. (1965). The visually evoked potential in twins. *EEG Jl*, **19**, 570

Elul, R. (1972). The genesis of the EEG. *Int. Rev. Neurobiol.*, **15**, 227

Emmons, W. H. and Simon, C. W. (1956). The non-recall of material presented during sleep. *Am. J. Psychol.*, **69**, 76

Empson, J. A. C. (1982). Slow potentials preceding speech. *Biol. Psychol.*, **14**, 271

Empson, J. A. C. (1983). Slow potentials preceding vocalization reconsidered. Presented at *1st Joint Conference on Experimental and Clinical Neurophysiology*, Burden Neurological Institute

Empson, J. A. C. and Clarke, P. R. F. (1970). Rapid eye movements and remembering. *Nature, Lond.*, **227**, 287

Empson, J. A. C., Hearne, K. M. T. and Tilley, A. J. (1981). REM sleep and reminiscence. In Koella, W. P. (Ed.), *Sleep 1980: Circadian Rhythms, Dreams, Noise and Sleep*. Karger, Basle

Ephron, H. S. and Carrington, P. (1966). Rapid eye movement sleep and cortical homeostasis. *Psychol. Rev.*, **73**, 500

Ertl, J. P. and Schafer, E. W. P. (1969). Brain response correlates of psychometric intelligence. *Nature, Lond.*, **223**, 421

Evans, C. R. and Newman, E. A. (1964). Dreaming: An analogy from computers. *New Scientist*, No. 419, 577

Evans, F. J. *et al.* (1970). Verbally induced behavioural responses during sleep. *J. Nerv. Ment. Dis.*, **150**, 171

Eysenck, H. J. (1967). *The Biological Basis of Personality*. Thomas, Springfield, Ill.

Fagen, J. W. and Rovee-Collier, C. (1983). Memory retrieval: a time-locked process in infants. *Science, N. Y.*, **222**, 1349

Feinberg, I. (1968). The ontogenesis of human sleep and the relationship of sleep variables to intellectual functioning in the aged. *Compar. Psychiat.*, **9**, 138

Fenwick, P. B. C. *et al.* (1977). Metabolic and EEG changes during TM: an explanation. *Biol. Psychol.*, **5**, 101

Foulkes, D. and Rechtschaffen, A. (1964). Presleep determinants of dream content: Effects of two films. *Percept. Motor Skills*, **19**, 983

Fowler, M. J., Sullivan, M. J. and Ekstrand, B. R. (1973). Sleep and memory. *Science, N.Y.*, **179**, 302

Freedman, R. R. and Sattler, H. L. (1982). Physiological and psychological factors in sleep-onset insomnia. *J. Abnorm. Psychol.*, **91**, 380

Freeman, G. K. (1978). Analysis of primary care prescribing – a 'constructive' coding system for drugs. *J. Roy. Coll. Gen. Pract.*, **28**, 547

Friedman, D. *et al.* (1975a). Cortical evoked potentials elicited by real speech words and human sounds. *EEG Jl*, **38**, 13

Friedman, D. *et al.* (1975b). The late positive component (P300) and information processing in sentences. *EEG Jl*, **39**, 255

Friedman, S. and Fisher, C. (1967). On the presence of a rhythmic, diurnal, oral instinctual drive cycle in man: a preliminary report. *J. Am. Psychoanal. Ass.*, **15**, 317

Gaillard, A. W. K. (1977). The late CNV wave: preparation versus expectancy. *Psychophysiology*, **14**, 563

Gaillard, A. W. K. (1980). Cortical correlates of motor preparation. In Nickerson, R. S. (Ed.), *Attention and Performance*, Vol. VIII. Lawrence Erlbaum Associates, New Jersey

Gaillard, A. W. K. and Perdok, J. (1980). Slow brain potentials in the CNV paradigm. *Acta Psychol.*, **44**, 147

Gaillard, A. W. K. and Verduin, C. J. (1985). Comparisons across paradigms: an ERP study. In Posner, M.I. and Marin, O.S.M. (Eds.), *Attention and Performance*, Vol. 11. Lawrence Erlbaum Associates, New Jersey

Gaillard, J.-M. (1975). Temporal organization of sleep stages in man. Presented at *2nd International Sleep Congress*, Edinburgh

Galambos, R. (1961). A glia-neural theory of brain function. *Proc. Natl Acad. Sci. USA*, **47**, 129

Galbraith, G. C. *et al.* (1970). EEG and hypnotic susceptibility. *J. Comp. Physiol. Psychol.*, **72**, 125

Gale, A. (1973). The psychophysiology of individual differences: Studies of extraversion and the EEG. In Kline, P. (Ed.), *New Approaches to Psychological Measurement*. Wiley, London

Gastaut, H. (1952). Etude electrocorticographie de la reactivité des la rythmes rolandiques. *Rev. Neurol.*, **87**, 176

Gerard, R. W. (1936). Factors controlling brain potentials. *Cold Spring Harb. Symp. Quant. Biol.*, **4**, 300

Geschwind, N. (1979). Specializations of the human brain. *Sci. Am.*, **241**, 180

Gevins, A. S. *et al.* (1979). EEG patterns during 'cognitive' tasks. 1. Methodology and analysis of complex behaviours. *EEG Jl*, **47**, 693

Giannocourou, M. (1984). Electrophysiological correlates of performance. Unpublished MSc Dissertation, University of Hull

Gillin, J. C. *et al.* (1979). Successful separation of depressed, normal and insomniac subjects by EEG sleep data. *Arch. Gen. Psychiat.*, **36**, 85

Globus, G. G., Gardner, R. and Williams, T. A. (1969). Relation of sleep onset to rapid eye movement sleep. *Arch. Gen. Psychiat.*, **21**, 151

Goff, W. R. *et al.* (1977). Origins of short latency auditory evoked potentials in man. *Prog. Clin. Neurophysiol.*, **2**, 30

Golla, F., Hutton, E. L. and Walter, W. G. (1943). The objective study of mental imagery. 1. Physiological concomitants. *J. Ment. Sci.*, **89**, 216

Goode, G. B. (1962). Sleep paralysis. *A.M.A. Arch. Neurol.*, **6**, 228

Goodenough, D. R. *et al.* (1975). The effects of stress films on dream affect and on respiration and eye-movement during REM sleep. *Psychophysiology*, **15**, 313

Griffin, S. J. and Trinder, J. (1978). Physical fitness, exercise and human sleep. *Psychophysiology*, **15**, 447

Grozinger, B. *et al.* (1974). Cerebral potentials during respiration and preceding vocalization. *EEG Jl*, **36**, 435 [abstract]

Guilleminault, C., Eldridge, F. L. and Dement, W. C. (1973). Insomnia with sleep apnea: a new syndrome. *Science, N.Y.*, **181**, 856

Halgren, E. *et al.* (1980). Endogenous potentials generated in the human hippocampal formation by infrequent events. *Science, N. Y.*, **210**, 803

Hansen, J. C. and Hillyard, S. A. (1980). Endogenous brain potentials associated with selective attention. *EEG Jl*, **49**, 277

Hansen, J. C. and Hillyard, S. A. (1983). Selective attention to multidimensional auditory stimuli in man. *J. Exp. Psychol.: Hum. Percept. Perform.*, **9**, 1

Harter, M. R. (1971). Evoked cortical responses to on- and off-set of patterned light in humans. *Vision Res.*, **11**, 685

Harter, M. R., Previc, F. H. and Towle, V. L. (1979). EP indications of size- and orientation-specific information processing: Feature-specific sensory channels and attention. In Lehmann, D. and Callaway, E. (Eds.), *Human Evoked Potentials: Applications and Problems*. Plenum, New York

Hartmann, E. (1968). The effect of four drugs on sleep in man. *Psychopharmacologia*, **12**, 346

Hartmann, E. (1976). Long-term administration of psychotropic drugs: effects on human sleep. In Williams, R. L. and Karacan, I. (Eds.), *Pharmacology of Sleep*, pp. 211–223. Wiley, New York

Hartmann, E. *et al.* (1971). Sleep need: How much sleep and what kind? *Am. J. Psychiat.*, **127**, 1001

Hassett, J. (1978). *A Primer of Psychophysiology*. Freeman, San Francisco

Hauri, P. (1966). Effects of evening activity on early night sleep. *Psychophysiology*, **4**, 267

Hauri, P. and Hawkins, D. R. (1973). Alpha-delta sleep. *EEG Jl*, **34**, 233

Hauri, P. and Olmstead, E. (1983). What is the moment of sleep onset for insomniacs? *Sleep*, **6**, 10

Haynes, S. N., Adams, A. and Franzen, M. (1981). The effects of presleep stress on sleep-onset insomnia. *J. Abnorm. Psychol.*, **90**, 601

Hebb, D. O. (1955). Drives and the CNS. *Psychol. Rev.*, **62**, 243

Heller, H. C. and Glotzbach, S. F. (1977). Thermoregulation during sleep and hibernation: Environmental Physiology II. *Int. Rev. Physiol.*, **15**, 147

Hennevin, E. and Leconte, P. (1971). La fonction du sommeil paradoxal. *Année Psychol.*, **71**, 489

Hernandez-Peon, R. (1966). Physiological mechanisms in attention. In Russell, R. W. (Ed.), *Frontiers in Physiological Psychology*. Academic Press, New York

Hillyard, S. A. and Munte, T. F. (1984). Selective attention to color and location: an analysis with event-related brain potentials. *Percept. Psychol.*, **36**, 185

Hillyard, S. A. *et al.* (1973). Electrical signs of selective attention in the human brain. *Science, N.Y.*, **182**, 177

Hishikawa, Y. (1976). Sleep paralysis. In Guilleminault, C., Dement, W. C. and Passouant, P. (Eds.), *Narcolepsy*, pp. 97–124. Spectrum, New York

Hopfield, J. J., Feinstein, D. I. and Palmer, R. G. (1983). Unlearning has a stabilizing effect in collective memories. *Nature, Lond.*, **304**, 158

Horne, J. A. (1981). The effects of exercise upon sleep: a critical review. *Biol. Psychol.*, **12**, 241

Horne, J. A. and Moore, V. J. (1985). Sleep EEG effects of exercise with and without additional body cooling. *EEG Jl*, **60**, 33

Horne, J. A. and Porter, J. M. (1976). Time of day effects with standardized exercise upon subsequent sleep. *EEG Jl*, **40**, 178

Horne, J. A. and Reid, A. J. (1985). Night-time sleep EEG changes following body heating in a warm bath. *EEG Jl*, **60**, 154

Hume, K. I. and Mills, J. N. (1977). Rhythms of REM and slow-wave sleep in subjects living on abnormal time schedules. *Wakng Sleepng*, **1**, 291

Israel, L. and Rohmer, F. (1958). Variations electroencephalographiques au cours de la relaxation. In Aboulker, P. *et al.* (Eds.), *La Relaxation*. Expansion, Paris

Isreal, J. B. *et al.* (1980). The event-related brain potential as an index of display-monitoring workload. *Hum. Fact.*, **22**, 212

Jasper, H. H. (1958). Report of the committee of methods of clinical examination in electroencephalography. *EEG Jl.*, **10**, 370

Jewett, D. L. and Williston, J. S. (1971). Auditory evoked far fields averaged from the scalps of humans. *Brain*, **94**, 681

Jones, H. S. and Oswald, I. (1968). Two cases of healthy insomnia. *EEG Jl.*, **24**, 378

Jouvet, M. (1963). The rhombencephalic phase of sleep. *Prog. Brain Res.*, **1**, 406

Jouvet, M. (1967). Neurophysiology of the states of sleep. *Physiol. Rev.*, **47**, 117

Jouvet, M. (1978). Does a genetic programming of the brain occur during paradoxical sleep? In Buser, P. and Buser-Rogeul, A. (Eds.), *Cerebral Correlates of Conscious Behavior.* Elsevier/North-Holland, Amsterdam

Kales, A. *et al.* (1966). Somnambulism: Psychophysiological correlates. *Arch. Gen. Psychiat.*, **14**, 586

Kales, A. *et al.* (1969). Psychophysiological and biochemical changes following use and withdrawal of hypnotics. In Kales, A. (Ed.) *Sleep Physiology and Pathology*, pp. 331–343. Lippincott, Philadelphia

Kales, A. *et al.* (1970). Hypnotic drugs and their effectiveness: all night EEG studies of insomnia subjects. *Arch. Gen. Psychiat.*, **23**, 226

Kamiya, J. (1967). Conscious control of brain waves. *Psychol. Today*, **1**, 57

Karacan, I. *et al.* (1971). New approaches to the evaluation and treatment of insomnia. *Psychosomatics*, **12**, 81

Karis, D., Fabiani, M. and Donchin, E. (1984). P300 and memory: individual differences in the Von Restorff effect. *Cogn. Psychol.*, **16**, 177

Keys, A. *et al.* (1950). *The Biology of Human Starvation.* University of Minnesota Press, Minneapolis

Klein, R. and Armitage, R. (1979). Rhythms in human performance: 1.5-hour oscillations in cognitive style. *Science, N. Y.*, **204**, 1326

Kleitman, N. (1927). Studies on the physiology of sleep: V. Some experiments on puppies. *Am. J. Physiol.*, **84**, 386

Kleitman, N. (1969). The basic rest–activity cycle in relation to sleep and wakefulness. In Kales, A. (Ed.), *Sleep: Physiology and Pathology.* Lippincott, Philadelphia

Kluvitse, C. D. (1984). The use of human event-related potentials in assessing mental work load and sleep loss effects. Dissertation in Industrial Psychology, Hull University

Kornhuber, H. H. and Deecke, L. (1965). Hirnpotential-anderungen bei Willkurbewegunger und passivess Beuregungen des Menschen: Bereitschaftspotential und reafferente Potentiale. *Pflugers Arch.*, **284**, 1

Koukkou, M. and Lehmann, D. (1968). EEG and memory storage in sleep experiments with humans. *EEG Jl*, **25**, 455

Koukkou, M. and Lehmann, D. (1976). Human EEG spectra before and during cannabis hallucinations. *Biol. Psychiat.*, **11**, 663

Kramer, A. F. (1985). The interpretation of the component structure of event-related brain potentials: an analysis of expert judgments. *Psychophysiology*, **22**, 334

Kuhlman, W. N. (1980). The mu rhythm: Functional topography and neural origin. In Pfurtscheller, G. *et al.* (Eds.), *Rhythmic EEG Activities and Cortical Functioning*, pp. 105–120. North-Holland, Amsterdam

Kupfer, D. J. (1976). REM latency: a psychobiologic marker for primary depressive disease. *Biol. Psychiat.*, **11**, 159

Kutas, M. and Donchin, E. (1977). The effect of handedness, responding hand and response force on the contralateral dominance of the readiness potential. *Prog. Clin. Neurophysiol.*, **1**, 189

Langford, G. W., Meddis, R. and Pearson, A. J. D. (1972). Spontaneous arousals from sleep in human subjects. *Psychonom. Sci.*, **28**, 228

Langford, G. W., Meddis, R. and Pearson, A. J. D. (1974). Awakening latency from sleep for meaningful and non-meaningful stimuli. *Psychophysiology*, **11**, 1

Lansing, R. W. (1957). Relation of brain and tremor rhythms to visual reaction time. *EEG Jl.*, **9**, 497

Lehmann, D. (1971). Topography of spontaneous alpha EEG fields in humans. *EEG Jl.*, **30**, 271

Levy, J. (1974). Psychobiological implications of bilateral asymmetry. In Dimond, S. J. and Beaumont, J. G. (Eds.), pp. 121–183. *Hemisphere Function in the Brain.* Wiley, New York

Lewis, S. A. (1969). Subjective estimates of sleep: an EEG evaluation. *Br. J. Psychol.*, **60**, 203

Libet, B. *et al.* (1983a). Preparation- or intention-to-act, in relation to pre-event potentials recorded at the vertex. *EEG Jl.*, **56**, 367

Libet, B. *et al.* (1983b). Time of conscious intention to act in relation to onset of cerebral activity (readiness potential). *Brain*, **106**, 623

Lindsley, D. B. (1951). Emotion. In Stevens, S. S. (Ed.), *Handbook of Experimental Psychology*. Wiley, New York

Lindsley, D. B. (1952). Psychological phenomena and the electro-encephalogram. *EEG Jl*, **4**, 443

Lippold, O. ᵂ. J. (1970). Origin of the alpha rhythm. *Nature, Lond.*, **226**, 616

Lisper, H. -O. and Kjellberg, A. (1972). Effects of 24 hours sleep deprivation on rate of decrement in a 10-minute auditory reaction time task. *J. Exp. Psychol.*, **96**, 287

Lister, S. (1981). A theoretical formulation of the effects of sleep loss. PhD Thesis, University of Hull

Loomis, A. L., Harvey, E. N. and Hobart, G. (1936). Electrical potentials of the human brain. *J. Exp. Psychol.*, **19**, 249

Loomis, A. L., Harvey, E. N. and Hobart, G. A. (1937). Cerebral states during sleep as studied by human brain potentials. *J. Exp. Psychol.*, **21**, 127

Loring, D. W. and Sheer, D. E. (1984). Laterality of 40 Hz EEG and EMG during cognitive performance. *Psychophysiology*, **21**, 34

Loveless, N. E. and Sanford, A. J. (1974). Slow potential correlates of preparatory set. *Biol. Psychol.*, **1**, 303

Lukas, J. H. (1980). Human auditory attention: the olivo-cochlear bundle may function as a peripheral filter. *Psychophysiology*, **17**, 444

Lukas, J. H. (1981). The role of efferent inhibition in human auditory attention. *Int. J. Neurosci.*, **12**, 137

Lukas, J. H. (1982). EEG correlates of sub-cortical gating. Presented at *2nd International Conference on Cognitive Neuroscience*, Queens University, Kingston, Ontario

McAdam, D. W. and Seales, D. M. (1969). Bereitschaftspotential enhancement with increased level of motivation. *EEG Jl*, **27**, 73

McAdam, D. W. and Whitaker, H. A. (1973). Language production: electroencephalographic localization in the normal human brain. *Science, N. Y.*, **172**, 499

McDonald, D. G., Schicht, W. W. and Frazier, R. E. (1975). Studies of information processing in sleep. *Psychophysiology*, **12**, 624

McGhie, A. and Russell, S. M. (1962). The subjective assessment of normal sleep patterns. *J. Ment. Sci.*, **8**, 642

McKee, G., Humphrey, B. and McAdam, D. W. (1973). Scaled lateralization of alpha activity during linguistic and musical tasks. *Psychophysiology*, **10**, 441

Malmo, R. B. (1959). Activation: a neuropsychological dimension. *Psychol. Rev.*, **66**, 367

Manaceine, M. de (1897). *Sleep: its Physiology, Pathology, Hygiene and Psychology*. Walter Scott, London

Manseau, C. and Broughton, R. J. (1984). Bilaterally synchronous ultradian EEG rhythms in awake adult humans. *Psychophysiology*, **21**, 265

Markand, O. N. *et al.* (1980). Brainstem auditory evoked potentials in chronic degenerative central nervous system disorders. In Barber, C. (Ed.), *Evoked Potentials*, pp. 367–376. MTP, Lancaster

Marxow, E. Fleischl von (1890). Mitteilung betreffend die Physiologie der Hirnrinde. *Zbl. Physiol.*, **4**, 538

Meddis, R. (1977). *The Sleep Instinct*. Routledge and Kegan Paul, London

Meddis, R. (1983). The evolution of sleep. In Mayes, A. (Ed.), *Sleep in Animals and Man*. Van Nostrand Reinhold, London

Meglasson, M. D. and Huggins, S. E. (1979). Sleep in a crocodilian, *Caiman sclerops*. *Comp. Biochem. Physiol.*, **63A**, 561

Mendels, J. and Hawkins, D. R. (1967). Sleep and depression. *Arch. Gen. Psychiat.*, **16**, 344

Merrick, A. W. and Scharp, D. W. (1971). Electroencephalography of resting behavior in cattle, with observations on the question of sleep. *Am. J. Vet. Res.*, **32**, 1893

Molfese, D. L. (1983). Event-related potentials and language processes. In Gaillard, A. W. K. and Ritter, W. (Eds.), *Tutorials in Event-related Potential Research*. North-Holland, Amsterdam

Monroe, L. J. (1967). Psychological and physiological difference between good and bad sleepers. *J. Abnorm. Psychol.*, **72**, 255

Moruzzi, G. and Magoun, H. W. (1949). Brain stem reticular formation and activation of the EEG. *EEG Jl.*, **1**, 455

Mukhametov, L. M. and Poliakove, I. G. (1981). EEG investigations of the sleep of porpoises. *Zh. Vyssh. Nerv. Devat.*, **31**, 333

Muldofsky, H. *et al.* (1975). Musculoskeletal symptoms and non-REM sleep disturbances in patients with 'fibrositis syndrome' and healthy subjects. *Psychosom. Med.*, **37**, 341

Murray, J. *et al.* (1981). Factors affecting the consumption of psychotropic drugs. *Psychol. Med.*, **11**, 551

Naatanen, R. (1982). Processing negativity: an evoked-potential reflection of selective attention. *Psychol. Bull.*, **92**, 605

Naatanen, R. and Gaillard, A. W. K. (1983). The orienting reflex and the N2 deflection of the event-related potential (ERP). In Gaillard, A. W. K. and Ritter, W. (Eds.) *Tutorials in ERP Research: Endogenous Components*. North-Holland, Amsterdam

Naatanen, R., Gaillard, A. W. K. and Mantysalo, S. (1978). Early selective-attention effect on evoked potential reinterpreted. *Acta Psychol.*, **42**, 313

Naatanen, R. and Michie, P. T. (1979). Early selective attention effects on the evoked potential. A review and reinterpretation. *Biol. Psychol.*, **8**, 81

Naitoh, P. and Townsend, R. E. (1970). The role of sleep deprivation research in human factors. *Hum. Fact.*, **12**, 575

Naitoh, P. *et al.* (1969). Modification of surface negative slow-potential (CNV) in the human brain after loss of sleep. *Psychophysiology*, **6**, 646 [abstract]

Naitoh, P. *et al.* (1971). Modification of surface negative slow-potential (CNV) in the human brain after loss of sleep. *EEG Jl.*, **30**, 17

Naitoh, P. *et al.* (1973). The effect of selective and total sleep loss on the CNV and its psychological and physiological correlates. *EEG Jl.*, *Suppl.*, **33**, 213

Nathan, P. W. (1969). *The Nervous System*, Penguin, Harmondsworth

Neville, H. J., Schmidt, A. and Kutas, M. (1983). Altered visual-evoked potentials in congenitally deaf adults. *Brain Res.*, **266**, 127

Nunn, C. M. H. and Osselton, J. W. (1974). The influence of the EEG alpha rhythm on the perception of visual stimuli. *Psychophysiology*, **11**, 294

Oatman, L. C. and Anderson, B. W. (1977). Effects of visual attention on tone burst evoked auditory potentials. *Exp. Neurol.*, **57**, 200

Oswald, I. (1957). The EEG, visual imagery and attention. *Quart. J. Exp. Psychol.*, **9**, 113

Oswald, I. (1959). Experimental studies of rhythm, anxiety and cerebral vigilance. *J. Ment. Sci.*, **105**, 269

Oswald, I. (1969). Human brain protein, drugs and dreams. *Nature, Lond.*, **223**, 893

Oswald, I. (1980). Sleep as a restorative process: human clues. *Prog. Brain Res.*, **53**, 279

Oswald, I. Merrington, J. and Lewis, H. (1970). Cyclical 'on demand' oral intake by adults. *Nature, Lond.*, **225**, 959

Oswald, I. and Priest, R. G. (1965). Five weeks to escape the sleeping pill habit. *Br. Med. J.*, **2**, 1093

Oswald, I., Taylor, A. and Treisman, M. (1960). Discriminative responses to stimulation during sleep. *Brain*, **83**, 440

Papakostopolous, D. and Fenelon, B. (1975). Spatial distribution of the contingent negative variation (CNV) and the relationship between CNV and reaction time. *Psychophysiology*, **12**, 74

Patrick, J. and Gilbert, J. A. (1896). On the effects of loss of sleep. *Psychol. Rev.*, **3**, 469

Peper, E. (1974). Problems in heart rate and alpha electroencephalographic feedback. *Kybernetik*, **14**, 217

Picton, T. W. *et al.* (1981). Auditory evoked potentials from the cochlea and brainstem. *J. Otolar.*, **10**, 1

Pitts, W. and McCulloch, W. S. (1947). How we know universals: The perception of auditory and visual forms. *Bull. Math. Biophys.*, **9**, 127

Plotkin, W. B. (1976a). Appraising the ephemeral 'alpha phenomenon': a reply to Hardt and Kamiya. *J. Exp. Psychol., Gen.*, **105**, 109

Plotkin, W. B. (1976b). On the self-regulation of the occipital alpha rhythm: control states of consciousness, and the role of physiological feedback. *J. Exp. Psychol.*, Gen., **105**, 66

Plotkin, W. B. and Cohen, R. (1977). Occipital alpha and the attributes of the 'alpha experience'. *Psychophysiology*, **13**, 16

Portnoff, G. *et al.* (1966). Retention of verbal materials perceived immediately prior to onset of sleep. *Percept. Motor Skills*, **22**, 751

Pravdich-Neminsky, V. V. (1913). Experiments on the registration of the electrical phenomena of the mammalian brain [in German]. *Zbl. Physiol.*, **27**, 951

Priest, R. G. (1978). Sleep and its disorders. In Gaind, R. N. and Hudson, B. L. (Eds.) *Current Themes in Psychiatry*, Macmillan, London

Purpura, D. P. (1959). Nature of electrocortical potentials and synaptic organizations in cerebral and cerebellar cortex. In Pfeiffer, C. C. and Smythies, J. R. (Eds.), *International Review of Neurobiology*, pp. 47–163. Academic Press, New York

Rechtschaffen, A. (1978). The single-minded and isolation of dreams. *Sleep*, **1**, 97

Rechtschaffen, A. and Kales, A. (Eds.) (1968). *A Manual of Standardized Terminology, Techniques and Scoring System for Sleep Stages of Human Subjects*. Public Health Service, US Government Printing Office, Washington, DC

Rechtschaffen, A. and Monroe, L. (1969). Laboratory studies of insomnia. In Kales, A. (Ed.) *Sleep: Physiology and Pathology*. Lippincott, Philadelphia

Rechtschaffen, A. *et al.* (1963). Nocturnal sleep of narcoleptics. *EEG Jl.*, **15**, 599

Regan, D. (1972). *Evoked Potentials in Psychology, Sensory Physiology and Clinical Medicine*. Chapman and Hall, London

Roffwarg, H., Muzio, M. H. and Dement, W. C. (1966). Ontogenetic development of the human sleep-dream cycle. *Science, N. Y.*, **152**, 604

Rosa, R. R., Bonnet, M. H. and Kramer, M. (1983). The relationship of sleep and anxiety in anxious subjects. *Biol. Psychol.*, **16**, 119

Rugg, M. D. (1983). The relationship between evoked potentials and lateral asymmetries of processing. In Gaillard, A. W. K. and Ritter, W., *Tutorials in ERP Research: Endogenous Components*, pp. 369–384. North-Holland, Amsterdam

Sassin, J. F., *et al.* (1969). Effects of slow wave sleep deprivation on human growth hormone release in sleep: preliminary study. *Life Sci.*, **8**, 1299

Schacter, D. L. (1977). EEG theta waves and psychological phenomena: a review and analysis. *Biol. Psychol.*, **5**, 47

Schafer, E. W. P. (1967). Cortical activity preceding speech: semantic specificity. *Nature, Lond.*, **216**, 1338

Shapiro, C. M., Catteral, J. R., Oswald, I. and Flenley, D. C. (1981). Where are the British sleep apnea patients? *Lancet*, **2**, No. 8245, 523

Shibasaki, H. *et al.* (1980). Components of the movement-related cortical potentials and their scalp topography. *EEG Jl.*, **49**, 213

Shucard, D. W. and Horn, J. L. (1973). Evoked potential amplitude change related to intelligence and arousal. *Psychophysiology*, **10**, 445

Snyder, E. and Hillyard, S. A. (1976). Long-latency evoked potentials to irrelevant, deviant stimuli. *Behav. Biol.*, **16**, 319

Sokolov, E. N. (1964). *Perception and the Conditioned Reflex*. Pergamon, New York

Spong, P., Haider, M. and Lindsley, D. B. (1965). Selective attentiveness and cortical evoked responses to visual and auditory stimuli. *Science, N. Y.*, **148**, 395

Starr, A. (1977). Clinical relevance of brain stem auditory evoked potentials in brain stem disorders in man. In Desmedt, J. E. (Ed.), *Auditory Potentials in Man*, pp. 45–57. Karger, Basle

Sullivan, H. S. (1953). *The Interpersonal Theory of Psychiatry*. Norton, New York

Surwillo, W. W. (1971). Human reaction time and period of the EEG in relation to development. *Psychophysiology*, **8**, 468

Surwillo, W. W. (1975). Reaction-time variability, periodicities in reaction-time distributions, and the EEG gating-signal hypothesis. *Biol. Psychol.*, **3**, 247

Sutherland, S. (1985). Left versus right. Review of Springer, S. and Deutsch, G., *Left Brain, Right Brain* (Freeman, London). *New Scientist*, No. 1461, 20 June, 32

Sutton, S. (1982). Musings on endogenous components. Presented at *2nd International Conference on Cognitive Neuroscience*, Queens University, Kingston, Ontario

Sutton, S., Braren, M. and Zubin, J. (1965). Evoked-potential correlates of stimulus uncertainty. *Science, N. Y.*, **150**, 1187

Szirtes, J. and Vaughan, H. G. Jr. (1977). Characteristics of cranial and facial potentials associated with speech production. In J. E. Desmedt (Ed.), *Language and Hemispheric Specialization in Man*. Karger, Basle

Tait, G. A. and Pavlovski, R. P. (1978). Alpha and the eye. *EEG Jl*, **45**, 286

Taub, J. M. and Berger, R. (1976). Effects of acute sleep pattern alteration depend on sleep duration. *Physiol. Psychol.*, **4**, 412

Taylor, J. (J d.) (1958). *Selected Writings of John Hughlings Jackson*, Vols. 1 and 2. Staple Press, London

Tebecis, A. K. *et al.* (1975). Hypnosis and the EEG: a quantitative investigation. *J. Nerv. Ment. Dis.*, **161**, 1

Tharp, V. K. Jr. (1978). Sleep loss and stages of information processing. *Wakng Sleepng*, **2**, 29

Tilley, A. J. and Empson, J. A. C. (1978). REM sleep and memory consolidation. *Biol. Psychol.*, **6**, 293

Tilley, A. J. and Wilkinson, R. T. (1982). Sleep and performance of shiftworkers. *Hum. Fact.*, **24**, 629

Treisman, A. M. (1969). Strategies and models of selective attention. *Psychol. Rev.*, **76**, 282

Velasco, M., Velasco, F. and Olvera, A. (1980). Effect of task relevance and selective attention on components of cortical and subcortical evoked potentials in man. *EEG Jl*, **48**, 377

Vogel, F. (1970). The genetic basis of the normal human electroencephalogram (EEG). *Humangenetik*, **10**, 91

Vogel, G. W. *et al.* (1975). REM sleep reduction effects on depression syndromes. *Arch. Gen. Psychiat.*, **32**, 765

Walker, J. M. and Berger, R. J. (1980). Sleep as an adaption for energy conservation functionally related to hibernation and shallow torpor. *Prog. Brain Res.*, **53**, 255

Walker, J. M. *et al.* (1978). Effects of exercise on sleep. *J. Appl. Physiol.*, **44**, 945

Wallace, R. K. and Benson, H. (1972). The physiology of meditation. *Sci. Am.*, **226**, 84

Walter, W. Grey (1953). *The Living Brain*. Duckworth, London

Walter, W. Grey (1964). The convergence and interaction of visual, auditory and tactile responses in human nonspecific cortex. *Ann. N. Y. Acad. Sci.*, **112**, 320

Walter, W. Grey *et al.* (1964). Contingent negative variation: an electric sign of sensorimotor association and expectancy in the human brain. *Nature, Lond.*, **203**, 380

Walters, W. J. and Lader, M. H. (1970). Hangover effects of hypnotics in man. *Nature, Lond.*, **229**, 637

Webb, W. B. and Agnew, H. W. (1964). Sleep cycling within twenty-four hour periods. *J. Exp. Psychol.*, **74**, 158

Weiskrantz, L. and Warrington, E. K. (1975). The problem of the amnesic syndrome in man and animal. In Pribram, K. and Isaacson, R. (Eds.), *The Hippocampus*. Plenum, New York

Weitzman, E. D. (1981). Sleep and its disorders. *Ann. Rev. Neurosci.*, **4**, 381

Wertheim, A. H. (1974). Oculomotor control and occipital alpha activity: a review and a hypothesis. *Acta Psychol.*, **38**, 235

Wertheim, A. H. (1981). Occipital alpha activity as a measure of retinal involvement in oculomotor control. *Psychophysiology*, **18**, 432

Wickens, C. D., Isreal, J. B. and Donchin, E. (1977). The event related cortical potential as an index of task workload. In Neal, A. S. and Palasek, R. F. (Eds.), *Proceedings of the Human Factors Society. 21st Annual Meeting*. Human Factors Society, New York

Wickens, C. *et al.* (1983). Performance of concurrent tasks: a psychophysiological analysis of the reciprocity of information processing resources. *Science, N.Y.*, **221**, 1080

Wieneke, G. H. *et al.* (1980). Normative spectral data on alpha rhythm in male adults. *EEG Jl.*, **49**, 636

Williams, H. L., Lubin, A. and Goodnow, J. J. (1959). Impaired performance with acute sleep loss. *Psychol. Monogr.*, **73**, 1

Williams, P. (1983). Psychotropic drug prescribing. *Practitioner*, **227**, 77

Williams, R. L., Karacan, I. and Hursch, C. J. (1974). *Electroencephalography of Human Sleep: Clinical Applications*. Wiley, New York

Wilson, J., Vieth, R. and Darrow, C. W. (1957). Activation and automation in right and left hemispheres. *EEG Jl.*, **9**, 570 [abstract]

Woodruff, D. (1975). Relationships among EEG alpha spectra, reaction time, and age: A biofeedback study. *Psychophysiology*, **12**, 673

Yingling, C. D. (1980). Cognition, action and mechanisms of EEG asymmetry. In Pfurtscheller. G. *et al.* (Eds.). *Rhythmic EEG Activities and Cortical Functioning*, pp. 79–90. North-Holland, Amsterdam

Yingling, C. D. and Hosobuchi, Y. (1984). A subcortical correlate of P300 in man. *EEG Jl.*, **59**, 72

Younger, J. Adriance, W. and Berger, R. J. (1975). Sleep during TM. *Percept. Mot. Skills*, **40**, 953

Zepelin, H. and Rechtschaffen, A. (1974). Mammalian sleep, longevity, and energy metabolism. *Brain Behav. Evol.*, **10**, 425

Zir, L. M., Smith, R. A. and Parker, D. C. (1971). Human growth hormone release in sleep: effect of daytime exercise on subsequent sleep. *J. Clin. Endocrinol.*, **32**, 662

Appendix: Program in BBC BASIC used to Average the AEP in Figure 1.5

```
>LIST
   10 MODE 4
   20 DIM PAD(300)
   30 DIM VEP(300)
   40 PRINT "Checking the brainwaves"
   50 MOVE 4.50
   60 FOR J=1 TO 300
   70 PLOT5.J*3.ADVAL(1)/64
   80 NEXT J
   90 INPUT"Brainwaves OK?".ANS$
  100 IF ANS$="N"THEN GOTO 40
  110 FOR J=1 TO 300:VEP(J)=0:NEXT
  120 CLS
  130 VDU 19.0.0.0:0
  140 INPUT"HOW MANY SWEEPS". SWEEP
  150 CLS:VDU 23.1.0:0:0:0:
  155 N=SWEEP
  160 REPEAT
  170 TIME=0
  180 SOUND 1.-15.69.20
  200 FOR J=1 TO 300
  210 PAD(J)=ADVAL(1)
  220 NEXT J
  230 FOR J=1 TO 300
  240 VEP(J)=VEP(J)+(PAD(J)/(N))
  250 NEXT J
  270 IF TIME<250 THEN 270
  280 SWEEP=SWEEP-1
  290 UNTIL SWEEP<1
  295 MOVE 4.50
  300 FOR J=1 TO 300
  310 PLOT5.J*3.VEP(J)/32
  320 NEXT
```

Selected Bibliography

Chapter 1

Brazier, M. A. B. (1961). *A History of the Electrical Activity of the Brain*, Macmillan, New York

Duckworth, D. (1976). *Understanding EEG: An Introduction to Electroencephalography*, Duckworth, London

Gale, A. and Edwards, J.A. (1983). The EEG and human behaviour. In Gale, A. and Edwards, J. (eds.). *Physiological Correlates of Human Behaviour, Vol 2: Attention and Performance*, pp. 99–128, Academic Press, London

Lippold, O. W. J. (1973). *The Origin of the Alpha Rhythm*, Churchill Livingstone, London

Regan, D. (1972). *Evoked Potentials in Psychology, Sensory Physiology and Clinical Medicine*, Chapman and Hall, London

Chapter 2

Lindsley, D. B. (1952). Psychological phenomena and the electroencephalogram. *EEG Jl*, **4**, 443

Nunn, C. M. H. and Osselton, J. W. (1974). The influence of the EEG alpha rhythm on the perception of visual stimuli. *Psychophysiology*, **11**, 294

Papakostopoulos, D. and Fenelon, B. (1975). Spatial distribution of the contingent negative variation (CNV) and the relationship between CNV and reaction time. *Psychophysiology*, **12**, 74

Plotkin, W. B. (1976). On the self-regulation of the occipital alpha rhythm: Control of states of consciousness, and the role of physiological feedback. *J. Exp. Psychol.*, **105**, 66

Chapter 3

Hillyard, S. A. and Kutas, M. (1983). Electrocortical signs of cognitive processing. *Ann. Rev. Psychol.*, **34**, 33

Loveless, N. E. (1983). Event-related brain potentials and human behaviour. In Gale, A. and Edwards, J. A. (eds.). *Physiological Correlates of Human Behaviour, Vol. 2: Attention and Performance*, pp. 79–98, Academic Press, London

Naatanen, R. and Gaillard, A. W. K. (1983). The orienting reflex and the N2 deflection of the ERP. In Gaillard, A. W. K. and Ritter, W. (eds.). *Tutorials in Event Related Potential Research: Endogenous Components*, pp. 119–142, North-Holland, Amsterdam

Chapter 4

Beaumont, J. G. (1983). The EEG and task performance: A tutorial review. In Gaillard, A. W. K. and Ritter, W. (eds.). *Tutorials in Event Related Potential Research: Endogenous Components*, pp. 385–406, North-Holland, Amsterdam
Geschwind, N. (1979). Specializations of the human brain. *Sci. Am.,* **241**, 180–199
Rugg, M. (1983). The relationship between evoked potentials and lateral asymmetries of processing. In Gaillard, A. W. K. and Ritter, W. (eds.). *Tutorials in Event Related Potential Research: Endogenous Components*, pp. 369–384, North-Holland, Amsterdam

Chapter 5

Dement, W. C. (1974). *Some Must Watch While Some Must Sleep*, Freeman, San Francisco
Meddis, R. (1983). The evolution of sleep. In Mayes, A. (ed.). *Sleep in Animals and Man*, pp. 57–106, Van Nostrand- Rheinhold, London
Oswald, I. (1980). Sleep as a restorative process; Human clues. *Prog. Brain Res.* **53**, 279

Chapter 6

Guilleminault, C., Dement, W. C. and Passouant, P. (eds.). (1976). *Narcolepsy*, Spectrum Publications, New York
Priest, R. G. (1978). Sleep and its disorders. In Gaind, R. N. and Hudson, B. L. (eds.). *Current Themes in Psychiatry*, Macmillan, London
Williams, R. L. and Karacan, Il (eds.) (1978). *Sleep Disorders: Diagnosis and Treatment*, Wiley, New York

Glossary

Acronyms and other abbreviations are defined in the text when first used, and their meanings should normally be clear, given the context. This glossary is provided to resolve any residual ambiguities or other sources of confusion, and as a handy source of reference.

ADC: Analogue–Digital Converter

A device that converts voltages into numbers – an essential first step in the computer analysis of the EEG.

AEP: Averaged Evoked Potential

The average of a number of evoked potentials – EEG responses associated in some way with a stimulus.

ARAS: Ascending Reticular Activating System

The nerve cells in the reticular formation which comprise the ascending pathways stimulating the thalamus and cortex, and controlling attentiveness and the level of arousal.

BP: Bereitschaftspotential

Sometimes referred to as the readiness potential. It is a ramp-like increase in negativity on the scalp surface, centred over the sensorimotor cortex, which precedes voluntary movements.

BRAC: Basic Rest–Activity Cycle

A short-term (approximately 90 min period in human adults) cycle in central-nervous-system functioning, which is independent of the alternation of sleep and wakefulness, but which periodically modifies both of these states.

CNV: Contingent Negative Variation

A waveform associated with a particular experimental procedure, in which a warning stimulus is closely followed (less than 3 s later) by an imperative stimulus, normally demanding a response. During the interstimulus interval the CNV or 'expectancy wave' — a ramp-like slow potential — develops on the scalp.

DC: Direct Coupling

Amplifiers which produce outputs directly in proportion to the input voltages are direct coupled. More usually, EEG amplifiers are AC (alternating coupled), and are insensitive to low-frequency activity to varying degrees expressed in terms of time constants (TCs).

EEG: Electroencephalogram

The electrical activity of the brain as measured from the surface of the scalp.

EMG: Electromyogram

The electrical activity of muscles.

EOG: Electro-oculogram

The electrical activity attributable to eye movement, normally recorded from above and below the eyes. EOG activity is largely determined by modulations of the corneo-retinal potential, as measured from the skin surface.

EP: Evoked Potential

Any EEg waveform associated with a stimulus, e.g. the so-called 'K complex' during stage 2 sleep, or, when a number of EPs have been collected and averaged, the AEP.

ERP: Event-related Potential

The average of a number of EEG waveforms associated with an event, which may be a stimulus (as in an EP), or the anticipation of a response (as in a BP), or the anticipation of a stimulus demanding a response (as in the CNV).

FP: Finger Plethysmograph

A device (frequently optical) which measures the volume of the finger, indicating both the tonic level of peripheral vasodilation and phasic (short-lived) changes which identify individual heart beats.

GSR: Galvanic Skin Reflex

The electrical activity of the skin, attributable largely to sweat-gland production, and responsive to autonomic arousal.

HR: Heart Rate

Measured in beats per minute (sometimes abbreviated to **BPM**).

Hz: Hertz

A measure of frequency – cycles per second.

N1:   First major negative component of the EP

(see Chapter 3).

N2:   The second major negative component of the EP

(see Chapter 3).

Nd: Processing Negativity

Negative EEG activity attributable to attentional processes
(see Chapter 3).

OR: Orienting Response

The psychophysiological changes (e.g. HR, FP, RR) accompanying the shift
of attention towards a novel stimulus.

P1:   The first major positive component of the EP

(see Chapter 3).

P2:   The second major positive component of the EP.

(see Chapter 3).

P300:   A late positive component of the EP

(see Chapter 3).

PCA: Principal Component Analysis

A set of statistical techniques aimed at identifying common factors underlying a series of numbers, which has been used in the analysis of event-related
potential components
(see Chapter 3).

REM or REMS: Rapid Eye Movement Sleep

A psychophysiologically distinct phase of sleep. See Table 5.1 and Figure 5.1 for its defining characteristics.

RR: Respiration Rate

Measured in breaths per minute.

SEP: Somatosensory Evoked Potential

Evoked potential elicited by electrical stimulation of the skin.

SWS: Slow Wave Sleep

In humans, slow wave sleep is conventionally defined as comprising stages 1 to 4 sleep.

TC: Time Constant

Defined as the time elapsed before 68 per cent of a square wave output from an AC amplifier has attenuated.

Index